T0362133

Global Perspective in Contemporary Orthognathic Surgery

Editor

YIU YAN LEUNG

ORAL AND MAXILLOFACIAL SURGERY CLINICS OF NORTH AMERICA

www.oralmaxsurgery.theclinics.com

Consulting Editor
RUI P. FERNANDES

February 2023 • Volume 35 • Number 1

ELSEVIER

1600 John F. Kennedy Boulevard • Suite 1800 • Philadelphia, Pennsylvania, 19103-2899

http://www.oralmaxsurgery.theclinics.com

ORAL AND MAXILLOFACIAL SURGERY CLINICS OF NORTH AMERICA Volume 35, Number 1
February 2023 ISSN 1042-3699, ISBN-13: 978-0-323-98787-5

Editor: John Vassallo; j.vassallo@elsevier.com
Developmental Editor: Jessica Nicole B. Cañaberal

Oral and Maxillofacial Surgery Clinics of North America (ISSN 1042-3699) is published quarterly by Elsevier Inc., 360 Park Avenue South, New York, NY 10010-1710. Months of issue are February, May, August, and November. Business and Editorial Offices: 1600 John F. Kennedy Blvd., Suite 1800, Philadelphia, PA 19103-2899. Periodicals postage paid at New York, NY and additional mailing offices. Subscription prices are $409.00 per year for US individuals, $785.00 per year for US institutions, $100.00 per year for US students/residents, $483.00 per year for Canadian individuals, $941.00 per year for Canadian institutions, $100.00 per year for Canadian students/residents, $535.00 per year for international individuals, $941.00 per year for international institutions and $235.00 per year for international students/residents. To receive student/resident rate, orders must be accompanied by name or affiliated institution, date of term, and the *signature* of program/residency coordinator on institution letterhead. Orders will be billed at individual rate until proof of status is received. Foreign air speed delivery is included in all *Clinics* subscription prices. All prices are subject to change without notice. **POSTMASTER:** Send address changes to *Oral and Maxillofacial Surgery Clinics of North America,* Elsevier Periodicals **Customer Service, 11830 Westline Industrial Drive, St. Louis, MO 63146. Tel: 1-800-654-2452 (U.S. and Canada); 314-447-8871 (outside U.S. and Canada). Fax: 314-447-8029. E-mail: journalscustomerservice-usa@elsevier.com (for print support); journalsonlinesupport-usa@elsevier. com (for online support)**.

Reprints. For copies of 100 or more, of articles in this publication, please contact the Commercial Reprints Department, Elsevier Inc., 360 Park Avenue South, New York, NY 10010-1710. Tel.: 212-633-3874; Fax: 212-633-3820; Email: reprints@elsevier.com.

Oral and Maxillofacial Surgery Clinics of North America is covered in *MEDLINE/PubMed* (*Index Medicus*), *Science Citation Index Expanded* (*SciSearch®*), *Journal Citation Reports/Science Edition*, and *Current Contents®/Clinical Medicine*.

Contributors

CONSULTING EDITOR

RUI P. FERNANDES, MD, DMD, FACS, FRCS(Ed)
Clinical Professor and Chief, Division of Head and Neck Surgery, Program Director, Head and Neck Oncologic Surgery and Microvascular Reconstruction Fellowship, Departments of Oral and Maxillofacial Surgery, Neurosurgery, and Orthopaedic Surgery and Rehabilitation, University of Florida Health Science Center, University of Florida College of Medicine, Jacksonville, Florida, USA

EDITOR

YIU YAN LEUNG, BDS, MDS, PhD, MOSRCS, FCDSHK, FHKAM
Clinical Associate Professor, Oral and Maxillofacial Surgery, Faculty of Dentistry, The University of Hong Kong, Hong Kong

AUTHORS

ALFRED G. BECKING, MD, DDS, PhD, FEBOMFS
Oral and Maxillofacial Surgeon, Department of Oral and Maxillofacial Surgery, Amsterdam UMC locatie University of Amsterdam, Amsterdam, Netherlands

YUNN SHY CHAN, BDS, MJDF
Department of Oral and Maxillofacial Surgery, Faculty of Dentistry, National University of Malaysia, Kuala Lumpur, Malaysia

AMIR ELBARBARY, MD
Professor, Department of Plastic, Burns, and Maxillofacial Surgery, Ain-Shams University, Cairo, Egypt

RIHAM ELDESOUKY, MD
Lecturer, Department of Plastic, Burns, and Maxillofacial Surgery, Ain-Shams University, Cairo, Egypt

MAIJA ELTZ, MD, DMD
Dr. Maija Eltz Institut für Kieferorthopädie, Vienna, Austria

MICHAEL D. HAN, DDS, FACS
Department of Oral and Maxillofacial Surgery, College of Dentistry, University of Illinois Chicago, Chicago, Illinois, USA

DONGMING HE, MD
Department of Oral and Cranio-Maxillofacial Surgery, Shanghai Ninth People's Hospital, College of Stomatology, Shanghai Jiao Tong University School of Medicine, National Clinical Research Center for Oral Diseases, Shanghai Key Laboratory of Stomatology and Shanghai Research Institute of Stomatology, Shanghai, China

FEDERICO HERNÁNDEZ-ALFARO, MD, DDS, PhD
Department Head, Institute of Maxillofacial Surgery, Teknon Medical Center Barcelona, Professor and Head, Department of Oral and Maxillofacial Surgery, Universitat Internacional de Catalunya, Sant Cugat del Vallès, Barcelona, Spain

VELUPILLAI ILANKOVAN, FRCS (Edin & Eng), FDSRCS (Edin & Eng)
Department of Maxillofacial/Head and Neck Surgery, University Hospitals Dorset NHS Foundation Trust, Dorset, United Kingdom

JOHAN JANSMA, MD, DDS, MSc, PhD, FEBOMFS
Department of Oral and Maxillofacial Surgery, University Medical Center Groningen, Department of Oral and Maxillofacial Surgery, Expert Center for Orthofacial Surgery, Martini Hospital Groningen, the Netherlands

LINGYONG JIANG, MD
Professor, Department of Oral and Cranio-Maxillofacial Surgery, Shanghai Ninth People's Hospital, College of Stomatology, Shanghai Jiao Tong University School of Medicine, National Clinical Research Center for Oral Diseases, Shanghai Key Laboratory of Stomatology and Shanghai Research Institute of Stomatology, Shanghai, China

TAKAHIRO KANNO, DDS, FIBCSOMS, FIBCSOMS-ONC/RECON, PhD
Professor and Director, Department of Oral and Maxillofacial Surgery, Shimane University Faculty of Medicine, Izumo, Shimane, Japan

CORNELIS KLOP, MSc
Medical Engineer, Department of Oral and Maxillofacial Surgery, Amsterdam UMC locatie University of Amsterdam, Amsterdam, Netherlands

TAE-GEON KWON, DDS, PhD
Department of Oral and Maxillofacial Surgery, School of Dentistry, Kyungpook National University, Daegu, Republic of Korea

YIU YAN LEUNG, BDS, MDS, PhD, MOSRCS, FCDSHK, FHKAM
Clinical Associate Professor, Oral and Maxillofacial Surgery, Faculty of Dentistry, The University of Hong Kong, Hong Kong

DION TIK SHUN LI BSc, DMD, MDS
Clinical Assistant Professor, Oral and Maxillofacial Surgery, Faculty of Dentistry, The University of Hong Kong, Hong Kong

GABRIELE A. MILLESI, MD, DMD
Assistant Professor, Department of Oral and Maxillofacial Surgery, Medical University Vienna, Vienna, Austria

KOMALAM MUGUNAM, BDS, MJDF
Department of Oral and Maxillofacial Surgery, Faculty of Dentistry, National University of Malaysia, Kuala Lumpur, Malaysia

JITSKE W. NOLTE, MD, DDS, PhD
Oral and Maxillofacial Surgeon, Department of Oral and Maxillofacial Surgery, Amsterdam UMC locatie University of Amsterdam, Amsterdam, Netherlands

ELAVENIL PANNEERSELVAM, MDS, MBA, FAM, FDS RCPS (Glasg)
Professor, Department of Oral and Maxillofacial Surgery, SRM Dental College and Hospital, Chennai, Tamilnadu, India

ANANTANARAYANAN PARAMESWARAN, MDS, DNB, MNAMS, MFDSRCPS, FDSRCS, FFDRCS
Professor, Department of Oral and Maxillofacial Surgery, Meenakshi Ammal Dental College and Hospital, Chennai, Tamilnadu, India

LAVANYAH PONNUTHURAI, DDS, MDS Prosthodontics (Kings College London)
Department of Restorative, Faculty of Dentistry, National University of Malaysia, Kuala Lumpur, Malaysia

BERNADETTE QUAH, BDS
Instructor, Discipline of Oral and Maxillofacial Surgery, Faculty of Dentistry, National University of Singapore, Resident, Oral and Maxillofacial Surgery, National University Centre for Oral Health Singapore, Singapore

RAMA KRSNA RAJANDRAM, MBBS, DDS, MFDS, MDS, OMFS (HKU)
Associate Professor, Department of Oral and Maxillofacial Surgery, Faculty of Dentistry, National University of Malaysia, Kuala Lumpur, Malaysia

MRUNALINI RAMANATHAN, MDS
PhD Resident, Department of Oral and Maxillofacial Surgery, Shimane University Faculty of Medicine, Izumo, Shimane, Japan

RUTGER H. SCHEPERS, MD, DDS, MSc, PhD
Department of Oral and Maxillofacial Surgery, University Medical Center Groningen, Department of Oral and Maxillofacial Suregry, Expert Center for Orthofacial Surgery, Martini Hospital Groningen, Netherlands

TIAN EE SEAH, BDS (Singapore), MDS (OMS, Singapore), FRACDS (Aus), FAMS (Singapore)Director
Director, TES Clinic for Face and Jaw, Visiting Consultant, Kadang Kerbau Women and Children's Hospital, National Dental Centre Singapore, Singapore General Hospital, Changi General Hospital

TIMOTHY JIE HAN SNG, BDS
Instructor, Discipline of Oral and Maxillofacial Surgery, Faculty of Dentistry, National University of Singapore, Resident, Oral and Maxillofacial Surgery, National University Centre for Oral Health Singapore, Singapore

ADAIA VALLS-ONTAÑÓN, MD, DDS, PhD
Attending Surgeon, Institute of Maxillofacial Surgery, Teknon Medical Center Barcelona, Associate Professor, Department of Oral and Maxillofacial Surgery, Universitat Internacional de Catalunya, Sant Cugat del Vallès, Barcelona, Spain

TOM C.T. VAN RIET, MD, DDS
Oral and Maxillofacial Surgeon, Department of Oral and Maxillofacial Surgery, Amsterdam

UMC locatie University of Amsterdam, Amsterdam, Netherlands

XUDONG WANG, MD
Professor, Department of Oral and Cranio-Maxillofacial Surgery, Shanghai Ninth People's Hospital, College of Stomatology, Shanghai Jiao Tong University School of Medicine, National Clinical Research Center for Oral Diseases, Shanghai Key Laboratory of Stomatology and Shanghai Research Institute of Stomatology, Shanghai, China

RAYMOND CHUNG WEN WONG, BDS, MDS(OMS), PhD, FAMS
Assistant Professor and Director, Discipline of Oral and Maxillofacial Surgery, Faculty of Dentistry, National University of Singapore, Senior Consultant, Oral and Maxillofacial Surgery, National University Centre for Oral Health Singapore, Singapore

HAO WU, MD
Department of Oral and Cranio-Maxillofacial Surgery, Shanghai Ninth People's Hospital, College of Stomatology, Shanghai Jiao Tong University School of Medicine, National Clinical Research Center for Oral Diseases, Shanghai Key Laboratory of Stomatology and Shanghai Research Institute of Stomatology, Shanghai, China

YONG WU, MD
Shanghai Wuyong Dental Clinic, Shanghai, China

CHEE WENG YONG, BDS, MDS(OMS)
Assistant Professor, Discipline of Oral and Maxillofacial Surgery, Faculty of Dentistry, National University of Singapore, Registrar, Oral and Maxillofacial Surgery, National University Centre for Oral Health Singapore, Singapore

MATTHIAS ZIMMERMANN, MD, DMD
Department of Oral and Maxillofacial Surgery, Medical University Vienna, Vienna, Austria

Contents

Currently, the wish to optimize facial esthetics—in the context of a dysfunctional occlusion or not—has become the main motivation for orthognathic surgery in many cases. In this context, considering that protrusive faces are advised more attractive and that the lack of skeletal support accelerates the aging process, orthognathic surgery will mostly involve a forward movement of the maxillamandibular complex.

Orthognathic surgery in asymmetric cases is challenging because of diversity and individuality. Clinical observations are of paramount importance and need to be systemically thorough. Three-dimensional diagnosis and virtual planning have been proven extremely helpful in facilitating treatment toward symmetry in difficult cases with increasing precision. Compared with orthognathic surgery in symmetric situations, asymmetries produce numerous pitfalls and provide opportunities for out-of-the-box procedures.

Bimaxillary protrusion is a unique dentofacial deformity trait that can exist in an individual as an isolated problem or in combination with other skeletal and dental-related issues. Orthodontist and oral and maxillofacial surgeons are often the main primary team involved in the management of bimaxillary protrusion. Clinical dilemma often exists as cases can either be treated orthodontically or may require a combination of orthodontic and skeletal segmental orthognathic surgery. This article aims to help clinicians improve their approach to management of bimaxillary protrusion by creating a classification based on the severity that can guide treatment selection.

Orthognathic surgery is an effective approach to correct vertical maxillary excess (VME), which is a common maxillofacial deformity and exhibits excessive vertical development of maxilla. This review summarizes different clinical features of total, anterior and posterior VME, as well as corresponding surgical managements guided by preoperative computer-assisted surgical planning. The virtual simulation will do favor to the final determination of individual surgical plans to achieve satisfactory outcomes. Finally, a typical clinical case will be presented to demonstrate the surgical management of VME.

In contemporary orthognathic surgery planning, the genium/chin constitutes an important part that contributes to the maxillofacial profile. The aesthetics of the lower face is affected by the position of the genium which makes reestablishment of genial morphology an essential component. It is hence necessary to evaluate the genium objectively on its individual merit, and any discrepancy is addressed accordingly. This review presents an overview of contemporary genioplasty techniques, their applications, and considerations on stability, osteosynthesis, complications, and the future developments.

Orthognathic surgery is a well-recognized method to correct dentofacial deformities. The main goal of orthognathic surgery is to improve soft tissue change. Soft tissue changes to the nose have been well documented. Simultaneous rhinoplasty during orthognathic surgery can be performed to correct existing inherent nasal deformities and also the unfavorable changes that arose from the maxillary surgery. Challenges for concurrent nasal surgery with jaw surgery include preoperative, perioperative, and postoperative which can be overcome with meticulous planning and experience. In complex cases, rhinoplasty can be staged in the last 6 months after the orthognathic surgery.

While primary cleft lip nasal deformity has been well described, secondary cleft lip nasal deformity reflects the combination of residual deformity that follows primary operative maneuvers and growth-related nasal distortions. Secondary cleft lip nasal deformities are further associated with underlying skeletal and dentofacial abnormalities along with soft tissue constriction adding to the complexity of the deformity and posing major aesthetic and functional challenges to the multidisciplinary care team. Definitive rhinoplasties are performed to address these deformities and improve the quality of life in cleft patients following skeletal maturity and ideally after all underlying skeletal discrepancies have been corrected by orthognathic surgery. Maxillary advancement with or without mandibular setback is often required after careful planning and orthodontic preparation. Patients with cleft lip benefit tremendously from definitive rhinoplasty irrespective of inevitable residual discrepancies that remain and adjuvant therapies could enhance the overall outcome.

An important aesthetic goal in orthognathic planning is to improve facial balance, harmony, volume, and symmetry. It is therefore logical that adjunctive aesthetic procedures become a part of the overall orthognathic treatment plan and that their possibilities are discussed with orthognathic candidates. Such procedures help to improve the final outcome of the orthognathic treatment and enhance patient satisfaction. Training and experience are of utmost importance when offering and performing aesthetic facial surgery. This article discusses various facial aesthetic procedures that can be combined with orthognathic surgery, to the patient's benefit, to help them become the most beautiful version of themselves.

ORAL AND MAXILLOFACIAL SURGERY CLINICS OF NORTH AMERICA

FORTHCOMING ISSUES

May 2023
Diagnosis and Management of Oral Mucosal Lesions
Neel Bhattacharyya and Donald Cohen, *Editors*

August 2023
Imaging of the Common Oral Cavity, Sinonasal, and Skull Base Pathology
Dinesh Rao, *Editor*

November 2023
Pediatric Facial Trauma
Srinivas M. Susarla, *Editor*

RECENT ISSUES

November 2022
Education in Oral and Maxillofacial Surgery: An Evolving Paradigm
Leslie R. Halpern and Eric R. Carlson, *Editors*

August 2022
Craniosynostosis: Current Perspectives
Srinivas M. Susarla, *Editor*

May 2022
Management of Melanoma of the Head and Neck
Al Haitham Al Shetawi, *Editor*

SERIES OF RELATED INTEREST

Atlas of the Oral and Maxillofacial Surgery Clinics
www.oralmaxsurgeryatlas.theclinics.com

Dental Clinics
www.dental.theclinics.com

THE CLINICS ARE NOW AVAILABLE ONLINE!
Access your subscription at:
www.theclinics.com

Preface

Global Perspective in Contemporary Orthognathic Surgery

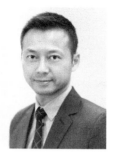

Yiu Yan Leung, BDS, MDS, PhD, MOSRCS, FCDSHK,
FHKAM
Editor

Dentofacial deformity affects patients' health, function, aesthetics, and self-esteem. The surgical correction of the deformed facial skeleton and the overlying soft tissue brings improvement to these important aspects of patients. In the past two decades, orthognathic surgery has further matured in the techniques as well as the treatment concept. Various forms of dentofacial deformity require specific considerations in surgical planning. There are some deformities that are more prevalent in certain ethnic groups, which require adjunctive procedures for their correction. There are newer concepts in aesthetic and the treatment protocol that are proposed, which could help to improve the overall treatment outcome and time. Technological advances in computer planning and three-dimensional printing have also brought orthognathic surgery to the next level. This issue focuses to describe the broad overview of the contemporary management of patients with dentofacial deformities from different parts of the world.

I thank Professor Rui Fernandes for the opportunity to contribute as an editor of this exciting issue.

I also thank Mr John Vassallo, Associate Publisher, and Ms Jessica Cañaberal, Continuity Development Editor, for their professional assistance throughout the editorial process. I am most thankful to all authors of the articles, who shared their expertise and experience in orthognathic surgery without reservation.

I dedicate this issue to all our patients, who entrusted us to correct their dentofacial deformities. Their confidence and trust motivate us as orthognathic surgeons to excel in our work to improve their faces as well as their quality of life.

Yiu Yan Leung, BDS, MDS, PhD, MOSRCS,
FCDSHK, FHKAM
Oral and Maxillofacial Surgery
Prince Philip Dental Hospital
34 Hospital Road
Sai Ying Pun, Hong Kong

E-mail address:
mikeyyleung@hku.hk

Aesthetic Considerations in Orthofacial Surgery

Federico Hernández-Alfaro, MD, DDS, PhD[a,b], Adaia Valls-Ontañón, MD, DDS, PhD[a,b],*

KEYWORDS

- Aesthetics • Orthognathic surgery • Maxillofacial surgery • Minimally invasive surgical procedures
- Imaging • Three-dimensional • Computed tomography • Cone beam

KEY POINTS

- When an "orthofacial" approach is embraced, surgical planning should focus to improve facial aesthetics, soft tissue support, temporomandibular joint, and upper airway volume, not only regarding occlusal purposes.
- The "Barcelona line (BL) is used to find the most aesthetic sagittal position of the maxilla, where a perpendicular true vertical line through the soft tissue nasion or so-called BL is traced.
- For diagnostic purposes, only a profile smiling picture with the patient in the natural head orientation position suffices to evaluate the relation of the BL with the upper incisor. In the context of surgical planning, the upper incisor should be positioned in or in front of the BL.
- Attractive faces are more protrusive than the cephalometric standards would like to accept.
- The forward reposition of the maxillomandibular complex involves beneficial aesthetic effects because the facial mask is tightened and therefore a reverse facelift is observed with subsequent improvement of nasolabial and labiomental folds and jowl areas.

INTRODUCTION

Orthognathic surgery (OS) indications have evolved substantially over the years due to a popular perception of surgery as a safe and predictable procedure, supported by the improvements in the surgical, medical, and orthodontic fields. Although correcting a dysfunctional occlusal and skeletal deformity used to be the key concern and almost exclusive therapeutic goal a few decades ago, nowadays it is clear that OS goes far beyond the mere correction of hard tissues. Its current uses comprise several functional indications, with the aim of correcting—a part from occlusion—also mastication,[1] phonetics,[2] temporomandibular joint disorders,[3] sleep-related breathing disorders,[4] and the avoidance of periodontal damage.[5]

Currently, the wish to optimize facial esthetics—in the context of a dysfunctional occlusion or not—has become the main motivation for OS in many cases.[6] Furthermore, the number of adult patients—not only young adults—who get involved in orthodontic or combined orthodontic-surgical therapy for both functional and/or aesthetic reasons is increasing steadily. It should be highlighted that when a dentofacial deformity (DFD) involves any skeletal hypoplasia of the lower and/or midfacial thirds, the lack of skeletal support accelerates the aging process, because typical unaesthetic facial features may appear precociously, such as poor projection of the lips, the early appearance of a double chin, and deepening of the nasolabial and labiomental folds, among others.[7]

Although the maxillofacial region is the key area of attention when planning an OS procedure, the

^a Institute of Maxillofacial Surgery, Teknon Medical Center Barcelona, Barcelona, Spain; ^b Department of Oral and Maxillofacial Surgery, Universitat Internacional de Catalunya, Sant Cugat del Vallès, Barcelona, Spain
* Corresponding author. Institute of Maxillofacial Surgery, Teknon Medical Center Barcelona, Barcelona, Spain.
E-mail address: avalls@institutomaxilofacial.com

Oral Maxillofacial Surg Clin N Am 35 (2023) 1–10
https://doi.org/10.1016/j.coms.2022.06.002

nose, the malar–midface, and the jawline regions are also critical determinants of overall facial esthetics, because the surgical creation of beauty requires the attainment of a correct balance between these three major facial prominences. Besides, the state-of-the-art treatment of DFDs through OS involves the comprehensive management of both the hard and soft tissues to correct any functional and aesthetic disharmonies of the maxillofacial complex.[7,8]

THE BARCELONA LINE: A DIAGNOSTIC AND SURGICAL PLANNING TOOL

Beauty is a subjective perception conditioned by individual and cultural preferences. Although facial beauty historically has been widely discussed, the contemporary attractive face entails protrusive, angled and defined lines. On the other hand, poor skeletal support of soft tissue manifests with premature facial aging.[8,9]

From this perspective, in 2010, the senior investigator described the "Upper Incisor to Soft Tissue Plane"[10] (**Fig. 1**) to trace the most aesthetic sagittal position of the maxilla in the context of DFD diagnosis and surgical planning. Nowadays, this tool has been renamed as "Barcelona line (BL) to ease its designation. In brief, after bearing out the natural head orientation (NHO) position of the head, a perpendicular true vertical line through the soft tissue nasion or so-called BL is traced. Then, the upper incisor should be positioned in or in front of the BL, providing upper lip support (based on adequate upper incisor angulation, or an orthodontically well-planned upper incisor position, with respect to the maxillary plane).

WORKFLOW PROTOCOL FOR ORTHOGNATHIC SURGERY VIRTUAL PLANNING

The BL protocol for OS virtual planning is based on a single cone-beam computed tomography (CBCT) scan (iCAT, Imaging Sciences International, Hatfield, PA, USA) of the head of the patient, with intraoral surface scanning of the dental arches using the Lava Scan ST scanner (3M ESPE, Ann Arbor, MI, USA) for subsequent fusion of the two data sets.[11] The data are primarily saved in Digital Imaging and Communications in Medicine format using three-dimensional (3D) software (Dolphin 3D Orthognathic Surgery Planning Software Version 11.8) for computer-assisted simulation surgery.

In addition, facial photographic records are obtained to complete the preoperative study

protocol. Patients are previously instructed by trained personnel to achieve the key points of photographic records for OS diagnosis and planning purposes: the patient breathing quietly without swallowing, sitting upright in the NHO position; indicating the patient to look straight ahead at a point in front of them at eye level (looking into a mirror); and the tongue in a relaxed position (**Fig. 2**).

For accurate virtual surgical planning, the BL protocol consists in a sequence of reproducible steps:

1. Definition of the desired final occlusion in the physical dental models.
2. Digital scanning of final occlusion and introduction of the 3D software for subsequent fusion with the CBCT data set.
3. Virtual head orientation according to the NHO position from the lateral resting facial picture. Then, this is considered the true horizontal line (see **Figs. 2**; **Fig. 3**).
4. Once the mandibular and maxillary osteotomies are designed, surgical repositioning of the maxillomandibular complex is virtually simulated. From the previously established final occlusion, maxilla and mandible are together positioned into class I.
5. The BL is traced: a true vertical line perpendicular to the true horizontal line based on the NHO position is drawn, crossing the soft tissue nasion.
6. The maxillomandibular complex is moved all together as a block with its upper incisor in or in front of the BL (see **Fig. 3**); it is extremely important that the upper incisor has the appropriate angulation or a well-orthodontically planned position with respect to the maxillary plane.
7. The dental and facial midlines are aligned, and the maxillomandibular complex is repositioned in all spatial planes (pitch, roll, and yaw) to set the virtual treatment objectives.
8. Clockwise or counterclockwise (CCW) rotation of the maxillomandibular complex is performed to achieve a proper occlusal plane.
9. Adequate projection of the chin is checked. In general terms, pogonion should be in or ahead the BL and the angle between occlusal plane lower incisor–pogonion should be around 90°. So, if necessary, a genioplasty is planned accordingly.
10. The exact vertical maxillary positioning is defined intraoperatively ensuring 2 to 3 mm of upper incisor exposure with relaxed upper lips.

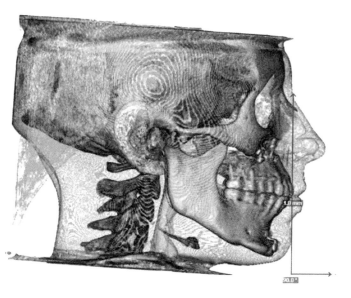

Fig. 1. "Upper Incisor to Soft Tissue Plane" or so-called "Barcelona line" (BL) to trace the most aesthetic sagittal position of the maxilla: after bearing out the natural head orientation, a perpendicular true vertical line through the soft tissue nasion or so-called BL is traced. Then, the upper incisor should be positioned in or in front of the BL.

FUNCTIONAL AND AESTHETIC ORTHOFACIAL IMPACT AFTER ORTHOGNATHIC SURGERY FOLLOWING THE BARCELONA LINE PROTOCOL

When an "orthofacial" instead of an "orthognathic" approach is embraced, surgical planning should focus to improve the outcomes in terms of facial

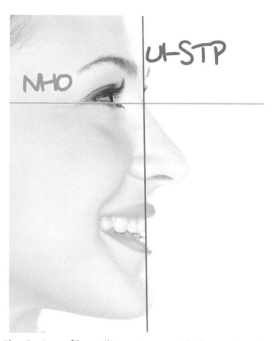

Fig. 2. A profile smiling picture with the patient in the natural head orientation to evaluate the relation of the "Barcelona line" with the upper incisor.

aesthetics, soft tissue support, temporomandibular joint, and upper airway volume, not merely considering jaws reposition for occlusal correction.

Although achievement of both functional and aesthetic goals has been the main objective of treatment planning of OS, most of the classical cephalometric analyses were centered on the false presumption that occlusion correction will result in ideal facial profiles.[12] However, from the early days, Peck[13] found attractive faces to be more protrusive than the cephalometric standards would like to accept. Since then, several investigators have described different analysis focusing on the maxillary sagittal forward positioning to achieve facial attractiveness.[10,14–16]

Regarding specifically the advantages of the BL protocol, we should mention that for diagnostic purposes, only a profile smiling picture with the patient in the NHO position suffices to evaluate its relation with the upper incisor, making clinical diagnosis easier and less invasive than radiologic analysis. Besides, the soft tissue Nasion point is not modified by surgery, which eases surgical planning and postoperative follow-up.

When using the BL protocol in Caucasian people, usually a forward maxillomandibular movement is required regardless of the initial occlusal situation of the patient or the amount of maxillomandibular discrepancy. Even most class III patients need some degree of mandibular advancement, as most patients present an underlying maxillary sagittal hypoplasia instead of a mandibular sagittal excess. Mandibular setback only appears to be necessary in a minority of

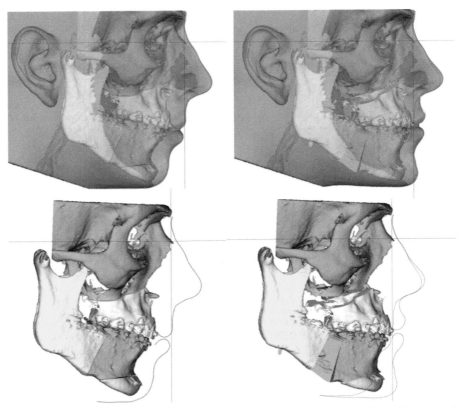

Fig. 3. Virtual planning according to the "Barcelona line," where the upper incisor is positioned in front of the BL.

cases, which are mostly coincident with a hemi-mandibular elongation or hyperplasia, an underlying acromegaly, or in cleft or syndromic patients.

In such cases where mandible setback is required, as it involves both functional and aesthetic drawbacks, CCW rotation of the mandible can be performed in some cases with a relatively prominent mandible. Mandibular CCW rotation can be also combined with setback to minimize the side effects of the latter.

On the other hand, mandibular advancement also presents other functional advantages over its setback, such as better long-term stability[17–19] and pharyngeal airway enlargement.[20] For the latter, forward movement of the maxillomandibular complex not only pulls forward the anterior pharyngeal wall but also enlarges the oral cavity and thus the tongue is better positioned anteriorly, and finally posterior airway space is less collapsed by the base of the tongue.[21,22] In this context, the maxillomandibular advancement has shown to be the most effective option for treating sleep-related breathing disorders in patients with an underlying DFD, with an 87.5% success rate.[4] Specifically, bimaxillary advancement and mandibular occlusal

plane changes by CCW rotation are the most significant contributors for upper airway enlargement[20] (**Fig. 4**).

ORTHOGNATHIC SURGERY IN THE AGING FACE

Facial aging process involves both soft (skin, fat, and muscles) and hard (facial skeleton) tissues. Although soft tissues migrate downward due to the effects of gravity and adipose and muscular tissue atrophy and wrinkles appear on the skin, the skeletal changes are generated by its resorption.[23,24]

Conventional antiaging surgeries were merely focused on skin pulling through face-lifting procedures. However, as Levine and colleagues[25] reported the importance of the role of bone in facial aging process, the concept of returning lost volume, mainly due to the loss of adipose tissue and bone resorption, to the face through fat grafting or fillers has become popular,[26–28] and a new philosophy based on facial skeletal expansion is now a matter of interest.[29]

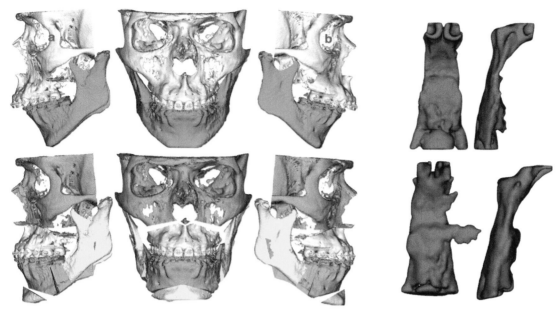

Fig. 4. Preoperative and postoperative CBCTs showing enlargement of the upper airway after orthognathic surgery planned according to the BL protocol with forward and counterclockwise movement of the maxillamandibular complex.

Therefore, in elder people, the forward reposition of the maxillomandibular complex involves beneficial aesthetic effects because the facial mask is tightened and therefore a reverse facelift is observed.[12,30–32] In other words, nasolabial and labiomental folds (**Fig. 5**) as well as the jowl (**Fig. 6**) may disappear without the necessity of performing a complementary face-lifting procedure.

Occasionally, the normal aging process entails the formation of a visible bulge in the area of the submandibular salivary glands that disrupts the planar and smooth surface of a youthful appearing neck. In these cases, the submandibular space can be suspended through an intraoral approach in the context of a bilateral sagittal split osteotomy (**Fig. 7**), improving the jawline contour, and thereby yielding a neck-rejuvenating effect.[33]

However, other procedures can be performed concomitantly with the OS when required, such as lipofilling, implants placement, bichectomy, or malar augmentation, among others.[28,34–36]

MANAGEMENT OF THE MAXILLARY SOFT TISSUE IN THE SAGITTAL DIMENSION

The 3D maxillary repositioning after Le Fort I osteotomy has different effects on the nasolabial region and the overall facial aesthetics. These

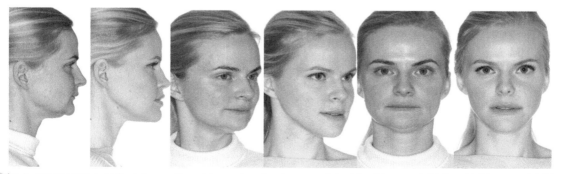

Fig. 5. Preoperative and postoperative pictures showing improved double-chin, nasolabial and labiomental folds area after orthognathic surgery planned according to the BL protocol with forward and counterclockwise movement of the maxillamandibular complex.

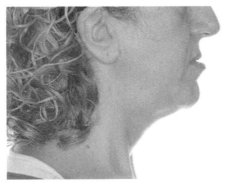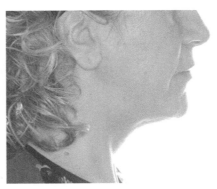

Fig. 6. Preoperative and postoperative pictures showing improved jowl area after orthognathic surgery planned according to the BL protocol with forward and counterclockwise movement of the maxillamandibular complex.

effects are related to the used surgical technique as well as to both the direction and magnitude of maxillary repositioning, and commonly include changes in the alar base dimension and morphology, the nasolabial angle, the position and shape of the upper lip, and the nasal tip projection.[37,38]

As previously mentioned, according to the BL protocol, most Caucasian patients with an underlying DFD undergoing OS require forward maxillary surgical movement. It may result upturning of the nasal tip, widening of the alar base, flattening and thinning of the upper lip, down-turning of the

oral commissures, and loss of vermilion of the upper lip. To minimize these side effects, the following pitfalls and recommendations should be considered:

- The degree of subperiosteal dissection and the degree of flap elevation may play an important role in changes in the perinasal soft tissues in this area. Therefore, a gentle subperiosteal dissection limited to osteotomy and fixation hardware placement area should be considered. Also, the pterygomaxillary disjunction should be performed through a

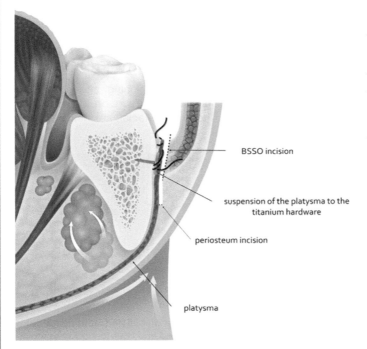

BSSO incision

suspension of the platysma to the titanium hardware

periosteum incision

platysma

Fig. 7. Suspension of the platysma of the upper aspect of the submandibular space to achieve a neck-rejuvenating effect. BSSO, bilateral sagittal split osteotomy. (*From* Hernández-Alfaro F, Guijarro-Martínez R, Masià-Gridilla J, Valls-Ontañón A. Jawline Contouring Through an Intraoral Approach in the Context of Bilateral Sagittal Split Osteotomy: A Proof-of-Concept Report. J Oral Maxillofac Surg. 2019;77(1):174-178.)

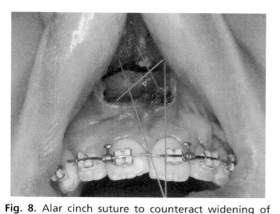

Fig. 8. Alar cinch suture to counteract widening of the alar base: inter-alar cross strap.

minimally invasive approach, such as the "twist" technique.[39]

- Most muscle insertions around the alar base area are detached during the conventional maxillary access, but the functions of the unaffected muscles with outer insertions remain unchanged. As the soft tissues are pulled by the remaining muscles, freeing of the facial muscles from the nasolabial area and the anterior nasal spine allows the muscles to be retracted laterally. Moreover, modifications of the traditional Le Fort I osteotomy that preserve the insertions of the perinasal musculature and the preexisting position of the anterior nasal spine and nasal septum through a subspinal osteotomy have been reported with excellent clinical outcomes.[40,41]

- In the same context, an alar cinch suture may counteract widening of the alar base: the fibroaerolar tissue of the base of the nose and the nasalis muscle are identified and with a suture it is pulled downward to the midline like a strap (**Fig. 8**).

- Finally, after muscular layer suture, a V–Y closure of the mucosa endorsed to counteract the detrimental effects of the Le Fort I osteotomy in the nasolabial region, as it thickens and projects the upper lip (**Figs. 9 and 10**).

SUMMARY/DISCUSSION

To sum up, current concept of "orthofacial" instead of "orthognathic" approach is preferable, because skeletal reposition of the jaws should not merely consider jaws reposition for occlusal correction but also to improve several outcomes in terms of facial aesthetics, soft tissue support, temporomandibular joint function, and preservation or enlargement of the upper airway volume.

For these purposes, the BL protocol has been proven as an adequate and predictable tool for diagnosis and surgical planning of DFD, which is used to trace the most aesthetic and functional sagittal position of the maxilla. In the diagnostic field, only a profile smiling picture with the patient in the NHO position suffices to evaluate its relation with the upper incisor, making clinical diagnosis easier and less invasive than radiologic analysis. On the other hand, surgical planning entails in most cases expansive maxillomandibular movements, regardless of the initial occlusal situation of the patient, or the amount of maxillomandibular discrepancy. Consequently, besides the good aesthetic results, it also improves soft tissue support providing an anti-aging effect and enlarges the upper airway volume, solving most sleep-related breathing disorders.

Finally, proper perinasal and upper lip soft tissue management after OS in terms of a subspinal osteotomy, an alar cinch suture, and a V–Y closure of the mucosa are essential to achieve better outcomes.

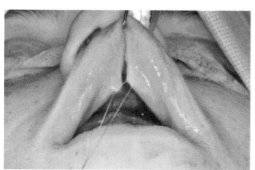
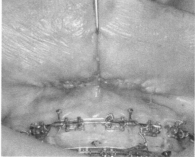

Fig. 9. V–Y closure of the mucosa to improve upper lip projection.

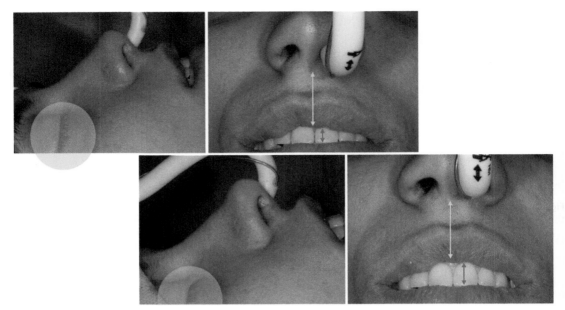

Fig. 10. Upper lip projection and length before and after V–Y closure of the mucosa.

CLINICS CARE POINTS

- Before starting surgical planning, ensure proper natural head orientation position of the virtual head.
- Use patient-tailored surgery instead of standardized surgeries according to patient's and surgeon's preferences.
- When deciding the sagittal maxillary position, keep in mind the volume and quality of the upper lip area.
- When pharyngeal airway is assessed, both volume and areas of constriction should be taken into account.

REFERENCES

1. Moroi A, Ishihara Y, Sotobori M, et al. Changes in occlusal function after orthognathic surgery in mandibular prognathism with and without asymmetry. Int J Oral Maxillofac Surg 2015;44(8):971–6.
2. Impieri D, Tønseth KA, Hide Ø, et al. Impact of orthognathic surgery on velopharyngeal function by evaluating speech and cephalometric radiographs. J Plast Reconstr Aesthet Surg 2018;71(12): 1786–95.
3. Ploder O, Sigron G, Adekunle A, et al. The effect of orthognathic surgery on temporomandibular joint function and symptoms: what are the risk factors? A longitudinal analysis of 375 patients. J Oral Maxillofac Surg 2021;79(4):763–73.
4. Giralt-Hernando M, Valls-Ontañón A, Guijarro-Martínez R, et al. Impact of surgical maxillomandibular advancement upon pharyngeal airway volume and the apnoea-hypopnoea index in the treatment of obstructive sleep apnoea: systematic review and meta-analysis. BMJ Open Respir Res 2019; 6(1):e000402.
5. Bernhardt O, Krey KF, Daboul A, et al. New insights in the link between malocclusion and periodontal disease. J Clin Periodontol 2019;46(2):144–59.
6. Belusic Gobic M, Kralj M, Harmicar D, et al. Dentofacial deformity and orthognatic surgery: Influence on self-esteem and aspects of quality of life. J Craniomaxillofac Surg 2021;49(4):277–81.
7. Posnick JC, Makan S, Bostock D, et al. Primary maxillary deficiency dentofacial deformities: occlusion and facial esthetic surgical outcomes. J Oral Maxillofac Surg 2018;76(9):1966–82.
8. Harrar H, Myers S, Ghanem AM. Art or science? An evidence-based approach to human facial beauty a quantitative analysis towards an informed clinical aesthetic practice. Aesthetic Plast Surg 2018;42(1): 137–46.
9. Mendelson B, Wong CH. Changes in the facial skeleton with aging: implications and clinical applications in facial rejuvenation. Aesthetic Plast Surg 2020;44(4):1151–8.
10. Hernandez-Alfaro F. Upper incisor to Soft Tissue Plane (UI-STP): a new reference for diagnosis and

planning in dentofacial deformities. Med Oral Patol Oral Cir Bucal 2010;15(5):e779–81.

11. Hernández-Alfaro F, Guijarro-Martínez R. New protocol for three-dimensional surgical planning and CAD/CAM splint generation in orthognathic surgery: an in vitro and in vivo study. Int J Oral Maxillofac Surg 2013;42(12):1547–56.

12. Mommaerts MY, Moerenhout BA. Ideal proportions in full face front view, contemporary versus antique. J Craniomaxillofac Surg 2011;39(2):107–10.

13. Peck H, Peck S. A concept of facial esthetics. Angle Orthod 1970;40(4):284–318.

14. Marchetti C, Bianchi A, Muyldermans L, et al. Validation of new soft tissue software in orthognathic surgery planning. Int J Oral Maxillofac Surg 2011; 40(1):26–32.

15. Arnett GW, Jelic JS, Kim J, et al. Soft tissue cephalometric analysis: diagnosis and treatment planning of dentofacial deformity. Am J Orthod Dentofacial Orthop 1999;116(3):239–53.

16. Marianetti TM, Gasparini G, Midulla G, et al. Numbers of beauty: an innovative aesthetic analysis for orthognathic surgery treatment planning. Biomed Res Int 2016;2016:6156919.

17. Politi M, Costa F, Cian R, et al. Stability of skeletal class III malocclusion after combined maxillary and mandibular procedures: rigid internal fixation versus wire osteosynthesis of the mandible. J Oral Maxillofac Surg 2004;62(2):169–81.

18. Proffit WR, Phillips C, Turvey TA. Stability after mandibular setback: mandible-only versus 2-jaw surgery. J Oral Maxillofac Surg 2012;70(7):e408–14.

19. Jakobsone G, Stenvik A, Sandvik L, et al. Three-year follow-up of bimaxillary surgery to correct skeletal Class III malocclusion: stability and risk factors for relapse. Am J Orthod Dentofacial Orthop 2011;139(1):80–9.

20. Giralt-Hernando M, Valls-Ontañón A, Haas Junior OL, et al. What are the Surgical movements in orthognathic surgery that most affect the upper airways? A three-dimensional analysis. J Oral Maxillofac Surg 2021;79(2):450–62.

21. Brunetto DP, Velasco L, Koerich L, et al. Prediction of 3-dimensional pharyngeal airway changes after orthognathic surgery: a preliminary study. Am J Orthod Dentofacial Orthop 2014;146(3):299–309.

22. Cabral MB, de Freitas AC, de Araújo TM, et al. Effects of chin advancement surgery in hyoid bone and tongue positions and in the dimension of the oropharynx. Dental Press J Orthod 2013;18(5):64–9.

23. Coleman SR, Grover R. The anatomy of the aging face: volume loss and changes in 3-dimensional topography. Aesthet Surg J 2006;26(1S):S4–9.

24. Fitzgerald R, Graivier MH, Kane M, et al. Update on facial aging. Aesthet Surg J 2010;30(Suppl):11S–24S.

25. Levine RA, Garza JR, Wang PT, et al. Adult facial growth: applications to aesthetic surgery. Aesthetic Plast Surg 2003;27(4):265–8.

26. Coleman SR, Katzel EB. Fat Grafting for Facial Filling and Regeneration. Clin Plast Surg 2015;42(3): 289–300, vii.

27. Ozer K, Colak O. Micro-autologous fat transplantation combined with platelet-rich plasma for facial filling and regeneration: a clinical perspective in the shadow of evidence-based medicine. J Craniofac Surg 2019;30(3):672–7.

28. Hernández-Alfaro F, Valls-Ontañón A, Blasco-Palacio JC, et al. Malar Augmentation with pedicled buccal fat pad in orthognathic surgery: three-dimensional evaluation. Plast Reconstr Surg 2015; 136(5):1063–7.

29. Rosen HM. Facial skeletal expansion: treatment strategies and rationale. Plast Reconstr Surg 1992; 89(5):798–808.

30. Lorente C, Hernández-Alfaro F, Perez-Vela M, et al. Surgical-orthodontic approach for facial rejuvenation based on a reverse facelift. Prog Orthod 2019; 20(1):34.

31. Sonego CL, Bobrowski A, Chagas OL, et al. Aesthetic and functional implications following rotation of the maxillomandibular complex in orthognathic surgery: a systematic review. Int J Oral Maxillofac Surg 2014;43(1):40–5.

32. Al-Hiyali A, Ayoub A, Ju X, et al. The impact of orthognathic surgery on facial expressions. J Oral Maxillofac Surg 2015;73(12):2380–90.

33. Hernández-Alfaro F, Guijarro-Martínez R, Masià-Gridilla J, et al. Jawline contouring through an intraoral approach in the context of bilateral sagittal split osteotomy: a proof-of-concept report. J Oral Maxillofac Surg 2019;77(1):174–8.

34. Raffaini M, Pisani C, Conti M. Orthognathic surgery "again" to correct aesthetic failure of primary surgery: report on outcomes and patient satisfaction in 70 consecutive cases. J Craniomaxillofac Surg 2018;46(7):1069–78.

35. Lazzarotto A, Franz L, Stella E, et al. Volumetric analysis of fat injection by computerized tomography in orthognathic surgery: preliminary report on a novel volumetric analysis process for the quantification of aesthetic results. J Craniofac Surg 2019;30(3):771–6.

36. Olate S, Uribe F, Huentequeo-Molina C, et al. Mandibular angle contouring using porous polyethylene stock or peek-based patient specific implants. A critical analysis. J Craniofac Surg 2021;32(1):242–6.

37. Bertossi D, Albanese M, Malchiodi L, et al. Surgical alar base management with a personal technique: the tightening alar base suture. Arch Facial Plast Surg 2007;9(4):248–51.

38. Magnusson A, Bjerklin K, Kim H, et al. Three-dimensional computed tomographic analysis of changes to the external features of the nose after surgically assisted rapid maxillary expansion and orthodontic treatment: a prospective longitudinal study. Am J Orthod Dentofacial Orthop 2013;144(3):404–13.

39. Hernández-Alfaro F, Guijarro-Martínez R. "Twist technique" for pterygomaxillary dysjunction in minimally invasive Le Fort I osteotomy. J Oral Maxillofac Surg 2013;71(2):389–92.

40. Hernández-Alfaro F, Paredes de Sousa Gil A, Haas Junior OL, et al. [Soft tissue management to control nasal changes after Le Fort I Osteotomy]. Orthod Fr 2017;88(4):343–6.

41. Mommaerts MY, Abeloos JV, De Clercq CA, et al. The effect of the subspinal Le Fort I-type osteotomy on interalar rim width. Int J Adult Orthodon Orthognath Surg 1997;12(2):95–100.

Management of Asymmetry

Tom C.T. van Riet, MD, DDS, Cornelis Klop, MSc, Alfred G. Becking, MD, DDS, PhD, FEBOMFS*,
Jitske W. Nolte, MD, DDS, PhD

KEYWORDS

- Orthognathic surgery • Facial asymmetry • Computer-assisted planning • Complications

KEY POINTS

- Outline the clinical assessment of facial asymmetry for orthognathic surgery, how to assess, and the role of posture.
- Differences and advantages of 3D virtual planning for orthognathic surgery in asymmetric cases compared with symmetric situations.
- Surgical techniques and additional procedures in treating facial asymmetry with orthognathic surgery.

INTRODUCTION

Management of facial asymmetry through orthognathic surgery can be a challenge. Not only the direction of asymmetry needs to be corrected, but also the shape and form of individual skeletal parts are frequently affected by remodeling and may require additional adjustments.

Restoration of asymmetry may be appointed for both functional and aesthetic reasons. A proper definition of asymmetry or symmetry from both the clinician's and the patient's point of view is key when starting any surgical journey. The influence of symmetry on facial attractiveness is subject to discussion and seems to be related to facial normality. Slight asymmetries in proportional faces can contribute to attractiveness, and symmetric disproportional faces can be considered unattractive.[1] Perception of these facial characteristics can differ between professionals and patients. Effective communication is, therefore, of utmost importance, and it might be useful to counsel patients with the use of a framework with categories of facial asymmetry.[2,3]

Etiology

Apart from the definition and proper communication about perception, knowing the origin of facial asymmetry is helpful when aiming for correction. It can be categorized in various ways, such as based on anatomic region, congenital versus acquired, origin of tissue, or neurologic background. The nature of asymmetrical tissue seems to be most important for clinical impact and treatment decision in orthognathic surgery and can be subdivided into dental, skeletal, and soft tissue features.

Soft tissue asymmetries are differentiated in separate components (eg, muscle, fat, skin, or all components) and expressed in overgrowth/undergrowth, and/or neurologic background. Masseteric hypertrophy, lipomatosis, or hemifacial hyperplasia reflect these different layers and do not adjust to orthognathic corrections as a matter of course. Impairment of any motor nerve, such as the marginal branch of facial nerve, might influence lip dynamics and cause canting of the lip, which is not possible to correct with orthognathic surgery. The clinician should be aware of the limitations of orthognathic surgery and address this during consultation, as part of expectation management.

Dental asymmetries, for example, in primary failure of eruption, can mimic skeletal asymmetries in extra-oral assessment and can be a pitfall when starting orthognathic treatment without simultaneous three-dimensional (3D) evaluation of the

Department of Oral and Maxillofacial Surgery, Amsterdam UMC locatie University of Amsterdam, Meibergdreef 9, Amsterdam, The Netherlands
* Corresponding author.
E-mail address: a.becking@amsterdamumc.nl

Oral Maxillofacial Surg Clin N Am 35 (2023) 11–21
https://doi.org/10.1016/j.coms.2022.06.013

underlying skeletal asymmetry or compensational changes.

Skeletal asymmetries are also the result of overgrowth or underdevelopment of the bony tissue, either congenital or acquired. The facial skeleton forms the basis of the resulting expression of the face, and should, therefore, be carefully studied at the beginning of the work up for a surgical treatment plan. The primary location of bony asymmetry should be detected, as well as any existing compensational changes.

Within the spectrum of skeletal facial asymmetrical disorders, the temporomandibular joint plays an important role. Forced bite or disc-displacement can mimic a (skeletal) asymmetry, which disappears when the mandibular condyles are guided properly into their fossa. This can be a challenge, especially in patients with persistent Sunday-bite or high muscle tension. It is advised to perform dynamic as well as static asymmetry assessments of the whole face, as differences can occur between them, which need to be addressed when planning corrective surgery.

A crucial factor in planning corrections for facial asymmetries is the presence or absence of progressiveness of disease. When ongoing changes are observed, no corrections should be performed until progression has ceased. Recognition of progression is key and clinicians should be aware that this can occur in both overgrowth conditions such as unilateral condylar hyperplasia (UCH) as in hypoplastic or degenerative disorders such as Parry–Romberg syndrome. Congenital asymmetrical conditions such as hemifacial hyperplasia, which grows proportional, or craniofacial microsomia, which is not progressive but can show increasing asymmetry due to continuous growth on the "normal" side, should be distinguished from this.

Detailed diagnostic criteria for all the asymmetrical overgrowth and undergrowth conditions are beyond the scope of this article. However, when assessing asymmetry, the abovementioned enumeration can be kept in mind. The following paragraphs will give a more detailed guidance towards clinical assessment, planning and pitfalls of orthognathic surgery in asymmetric patients.

CLINICAL ASSESSMENT
Challenges in the Determination of Facial Asymmetry

With regard to its clinical assessment, facial asymmetry can be considered a variation in size, shape or arrangement of facial landmarks between 2 sides of the face, split by an imaginary facial midline. A reliable determination of this facial midline is essential in every attempt to assess facial symmetry, but it also represents an important issue, as frequently used reference points might not represent the true median sagittal plane.[4]

Instead of being directional, asymmetric features can occur in the lower, mid-and upper parts of the face "fluctuating" between the left and right sides. As explained in the etiology section, they can originate from skeletal, soft tissue, dental and functional structures. As the degree of asymmetry can differ between soft tissues and underlying hard tissues, they can potentially mask or compensate for any existing asymmetry in another structure.

The most frequently used techniques for the clinical assessment of facial asymmetry make use of the natural head position (NHP).[5] However, postural compensations for facial asymmetry, for example, by tilting the head slightly, are frequent and can seriously hinder clinicians in correctly characterizing facial imbalances.[6]

Qualitative Evaluation of Asymmetries

The foremost step in assessing facial asymmetry is direct clinical examination. While a complete instruction on the clinical examination of the face falls outside the scope of this article, some clinical tips in the light of asymmetry are supplied. At first, a visual and palpable inspection of facial structures and contours should be performed. During this examination, it is important to keep the patients' face completely unveiled. It can be beneficial to compare important midline landmarks (ie, soft-tissue glabella, nasal tip, and pogonion) to the true facial midline, either from standing behind the patient or from a worm's-eye perspective. In challenging cases, it can be of additional value to "block" parts of the face with a piece of paper and mark the landmarks of the lower, mid, and upper facial parts individually, with the use of a marker, before doing a comparison to the facial midline. Another technique to evaluate an asymmetric lower part of the face is to guide the mandible laterally to align the chin with the facial midline and to evaluate subsequent occlusal and facial changes.[7] The orientation of the occlusal plane can be evaluated through an extra-oral examination by holding a spatula between the canines and compare its orientation with the interpupillary line. It is essential to ensure a NHP in this step, which is further explained in the next paragraph on 3D planning. Spatulas with a stepwise increase in thickness on one side can be potentially useful to quantify any existing differences.

Intraorally, traditional occlusal traits should be evaluated. Special attention should be paid to any occlusal interferences that might cause functional mandibular shifts and therefore induce or mimic mandibular asymmetry. Next to the dental midlines, it can be of additional value to measure the amount of gingival show in the maxilla on both sides separately.

Quantitative evaluation of asymmetries

Although clinical examination is essential to evaluate qualitative facial asymmetry, it is less suitable for its quantification. Digital photography can have additional value to the clinical examination, but quantification is not possible as there is geometric distortion due to magnification errors. To quantify and deepen the evaluation of facial asymmetry, several techniques have been developed using laser surface scanning technology,[8] 3D-stereophotogrammetry[9,10] and 3D radiographic imaging. One of the major advantages of quantification is the possibility to monitor asymmetries during follow-up examinations. Despite their advantages, these techniques should be considered supportive of the diagnostic process and not as a replacement for a comprehensive clinical examination.

Three-dimensional stereophotogrammetry can be used to objectify and quantify facial soft-tissue asymmetries in all 3 planes with several different techniques. The face can be mirrored using an arbitrary plane outside the face, followed by cranial base registration, which eliminates the problem of identifying a midsagittal plane.[9] In another technique, the face is compared with an aligned perfect symmetric dummy.[10] These methods do not need exposure to radiation, are low-cost, fast and landmark-independent. The latter is important as the traditional landmark-based evaluation of asymmetry, also in 3 dimensions, does not take entire facial structures into account and performs less than surface-based methods.[11]

For skeletal asymmetry assessment, the use of traditional landmark-based radiography (two-dimensional) has long been deemed insufficiently reliable.[12] To evaluate the complex nature of skeletal facial asymmetry, 3D evaluation is essential. Due to improvement in (cone-beam) radiological technologies, soft tissues can also be reliably evaluated with these techniques. With different methods such as surface area, distance, or volumetric measurements, morphologic asymmetries can be evaluated in detail.[13]

Next-Generation Techniques

Machine learning techniques can be particularly useful to understand and analyze complex data with many variables. Modern learning techniques in orthognathic surgery are explored in many ways, for example, to assess the impact of orthognathic treatment on facial attractiveness and automated cephalometric landmark detection in 3D imaging.[14–16] These techniques can be potentially useful for objectively determining facial asymmetry. Modern computer vision algorithms have been used to automatically process 3D images and construct high-dimensional statistical models of the facial shape.[17] In other scientific efforts, an algorithm was designed that aids in the determination of the facial midline[18] and allowing for real-time dynamic analysis of facial asymmetry.[19] Despite the fact that these techniques are still in a developmental phase, they are specifically developed to overcome some of the mentioned difficulties in the assessment of facial asymmetry. It can be expected that it will significantly change the way we assess facial asymmetry in the next few years.

3D VIRTUAL PLANNING
Head Position for Planning

Determining the head position for planning (HPP) is fundamental for 3D virtual planning. The HPP might be the patient's NHP, but these are not identical by definition. Usually, the HPP is established using a combination of clinical assessment and clinical photographs. During the clinical assessment, important parameters to evaluate are the interpupillary line, the maxillary midline deviation compared with the facial midline, and the dental show at rest and smiling. Clinical photographs should be obtained at rest and smiling, in both frontal and lateral views.

The approach for determining the frontal HPP depends on the degree of asymmetry in the midface and upper face areas. In case of predominantly lower face asymmetry (eg, UCH), the HPP can often be established by assuming a horizontal interpupillary line and by using the symmetry of the upper midface and forehead (**Fig. 1**). Then, the midsagittal plane is defined through the center of the nose bridge. The resulting midline deviation of the maxilla should be compared with the clinical measurements. If there is no consensus among these 2, either one of the head positions is chosen, or a compromise between the 2 is sought.

In case of extensive facial asymmetry (eg, craniofacial microsomia with orbital involvement), the interpupillary line and the symmetry of the midface and upper face areas are not reliable. In such cases, the NHP of the patient can be used for planning (**Fig. 2**). To find a reproducible NHP, clinical photographs should be obtained on multiple

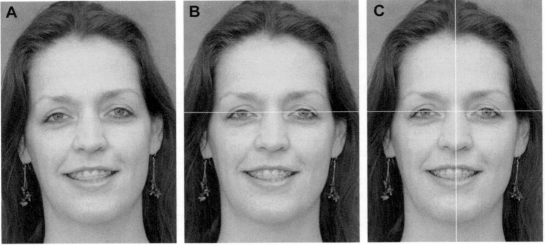

Fig. 1. Frontal head position for planning in case of predominantly lower face asymmetry. (*A*) Baseline clinical photograph. (*B*) *Rotation of the patient's posture is corrected* by setting the interpupillary line horizontal. (*C*) Midsagittal plane is set through the center of the nose bridge.

occasions. The average head position on these photographs should be used as HPP. Using a mirror can assist the patient in finding the most natural and comfortable head position. The rotation of the camera should be standardized by using a tripod or by having a true vertical line visible on the photographs, such as a vertical laser line.

The bottom line for establishing the frontal HPP for asymmetric patients is as follows. In case of predominantly lower face asymmetry, a correction is applied for the *rotation of the patient's posture*, using the symmetry of the upper face. In case of extensive facial asymmetry, a correction is applied for the *rotation of the camera*, using a true vertical line.

The lateral HPP can be established by either using a standardized head position, such as the commonly used Frankfurt horizontal plane, or by using the patient's NHP on clinical photographs (**Fig. 3**).

3D Virtual Planning

Contemporary orthognathic planning relies on a high-quality computed tomography (CT) or cone-beam CT (CBCT) scan. A high-quality scan implies the absence of movement artifacts (**Fig. 4**A) and adequate condylar seating using the retruded contact position (**Fig. 4**B). 3D virtual planning is conducted in software that allows for creating a hard tissue and soft tissue model of the patient. Due

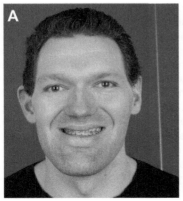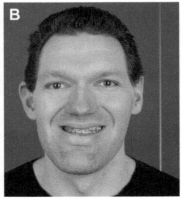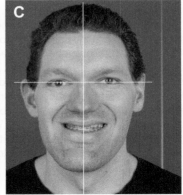

Fig. 2. Frontal head position for planning in case of extensive facial asymmetry. (*A*) Baseline clinical photograph. (*B*) *Rotation of the camera is corrected* using a true vertical line (*laser line*). (*C*) Midsagittal plane is set through the center of the nose bridge; the interpupillary line is not necessarily horizontal.

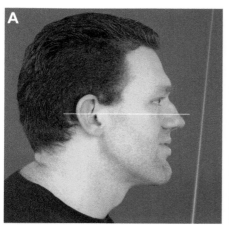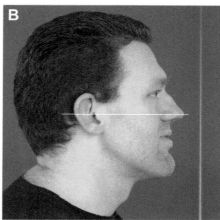

Fig. 3. Establishing the lateral head position for planning. (*A*) Using the Frankfurter horizontal plane. (*B*) Using the patient's natural head position.

to the density of enamel and the presence of dental restorations, the dentition is rendered of insufficient quality in the hard tissue model. Fusing high-quality dental models into the hard tissue model is, therefore, an indispensable feature in these software packages. Dental models can be obtained by intraoral scanning or by acquiring a CT scan of traditional stone cast models. Setting the desired postoperative occlusion is the next step, so that the bimaxillary complex can be translated and rotated as a unit. Determining the postoperative occlusion can be conducted either on the physical dental casts or with the use of a virtual occlusion tool.

In the 3D world we live in, there are 6° of freedom; 3 translations consisting of (1) forward-backward, (2) left-right, and (3) up–down movements and thee rotations consisting of (1) roll (rotation about the antero-posterior axis), (2) pitch

(rotation about the left–right axis), and (3) yaw (rotation about the vertical axis). The rotations are shown in **Fig. 5** for further explanation. The left–right shift, roll, and yaw are degrees of freedom that are governed by symmetry. The other 3, forward–backward shift, up–down shift, and pitch, influence important esthetic parameters such as the profile, chin projection, and dental show. A virtual orthognathic planning of an asymmetric case is demonstrated in **Fig. 5**.

The left–right shift should be corrected according to the HPP that was established; the maxillary incisor midpoint should align with the patient's midsagittal plane. For rotations, the maxillary incisor midpoint is commonly used as a rotation pivot. The roll-correction is controlled by the occlusal cant and the symmetry of the chin. The yaw-correction is often a compromise between the symmetry of the upper dentition, lower

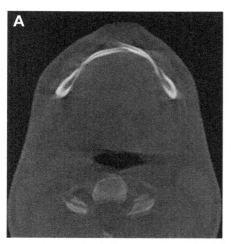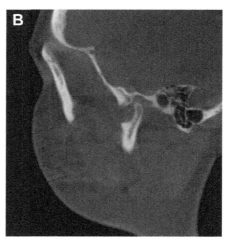

Fig. 4. Two major factors that influence scan quality. (*A*) Movement artifacts. (*B*) Insufficient condylar seating due to misrecording of the retruded contact position.

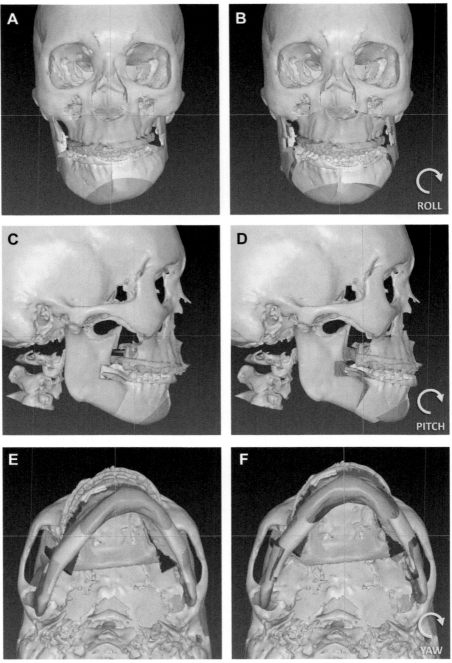

Fig. 5. 3D virtual bimaxillary osteotomy and genioplasty planning of an asymmetric case. (*A, C, E*) Preoperative situation. (*B, D, F*) Planned situation. The roll, pitch, and yaw parameters are demonstrated.

dentition, and symmetry on the bony level. Cephalometric landmarks can be of significant benefit in 3D virtual planning, as they provide objective measurements.

In case of remaining asymmetry in the chin area, a genioplasty can be considered, for which a 3D virtual planning is advised (see **Fig. 5**). The genioplasty can be performed manually, or by using 3D printed cutting and drilling guides in combination with stock plates. Alternatively, a titanium patient-specific implant may be designed and manufactured, potentially leading to more predictive and accurate results. Symmetry in the proximal segments (eg, unilateral or intergonial width)

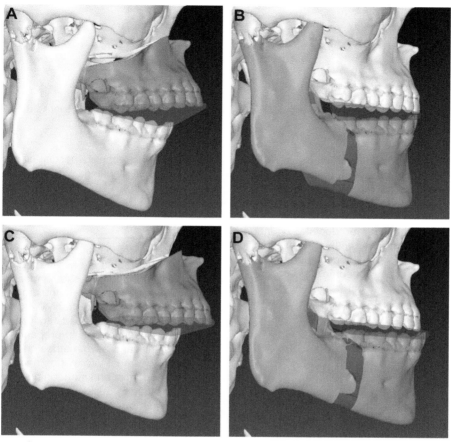

Fig. 6. (*A*) Interference of the maxillary and mandibular dentition can be solved by the autorotation of the mandible, but this introduces additional inaccuracy and excessive splint thickness. (*B*) This issue is resolved by the mandible-first approach. (*C*) Excessive overhang of the maxilla-first splint. (*D*) This issue is resolved by switching to mandible-first.

is difficult to correct during orthognathic surgery and is common in patients with UCH. This is frequently treated secondarily. For the augmentation of the underprojected side, correction can be considered using a stock contouring implant, a patient-specific implant, or a soft tissue treatment such as lipofilling. Reduction of the overprojected side can be achieved by using 3D printed cutting guides. The use of virtual planning is advised, whether or not a patient-specific solution is used for treatment.

Transferring the Planning to Surgery

In most asymmetric orthognathic cases, the 3D planning is transferred into surgical steps with 3D printed dental splints. The final splint determines the postoperative occlusion. The intermediate splint transfers one jaw into the planned position and retains the other jaw in the original position, ensuring reference at all times. Most surgeons

prefer a typical order of surgery in which either the maxilla or mandible is operated on first. The maxilla-first approach can be considered the classic approach, but in asymmetric patients, several reasons exist to choose mandible-first instead.

In asymmetric patients, the condylar seating may be inadequate, especially in cases of CFM, postankylosis, or postcondylectomy. In such cases, the mandible-first approach might be favored over the maxilla-first approach. Operating the mandible first may also be preferred in bimaxillary procedures with multi-piece Le Fort I osteotomies. A third reason to switch the order of surgery would be the interference of the maxillary and mandibular dentition in the intermediate position. This can be solved by the autorotation of the mandible, but in general, this introduces additional inaccuracy and adds to the splint thickness in the frontal area (**Fig. 6**A, B). In this case, the mandible-first approach is suggested. Another reason to

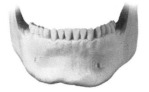 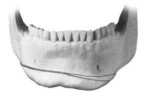 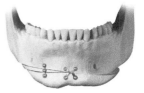

Fig. 7. Propeller wedge technique to correct an asymmetric chin; the wedge is swapped over to the contralateral side and fixed.

perform the surgery mandible-first, which is not strictly asymmetry-related, is an excessive thickness or overhang of the intermediate splint, leading to an unstable situation during intermaxillary fixation (**Fig. 6**C, D). When the condylar seating is generally unreliable, irreproducible, or inadequate, splintless surgery with patient-specific guides and implants should be considered. Splintless surgery may certainly become state-of-the-art for orthognathic surgery, but is currently associated with excessive costs compared with conventional splints.

SPECIFIC CONSIDERATIONS IN ORTHOGNATHIC SURGERY WITH ASYMMETRY

Current orthognathic surgery planning for asymmetries cannot be conducted accurately without 3D virtual planning. Especially for the virtual repositioning of the maxilla in 3 dimensions with translations, yaw, roll, and pitch, which is the cornerstone of the surgical plan. Subsequently, the mandible is planned toward maximal occlusion after which further fine-tuning of the chin, mandibular angles, and zygomatic bone(s) is performed to virtually correct asymmetries, leading toward an optimal plan. Treatment toward optimal bony and dental symmetry is not necessarily followed by corresponding soft tissue symmetry. Additionally, soft tissue correction may be necessary and is ideally sequenced after bony correction.

Especially in gross asymmetries, challenges will be present in which even contradictory movements of bone may be anticipated. Correcting the yaw in the maxilla may either correct or rather introduce asymmetric paranasal fullness. Coordinating the maxillary dental arch with the bony base in the maxilla is mandatory in this respect, but unfortunately not always possible, as in severe cleft or unilateral microsomia cases. Correcting a yaw of the maxilla will also influence, for better or worse, the flaring of mandibular angles, lower border, and chin position. Correcting a roll in de maxilla will influence the vertical position of the lower border of the mandible, and the roll in the

chin area, again either beneficial or contradictory toward an ideal planning.

Technical Topics in Orthognathic Surgery for Asymmetry

1. Orthodontics. In orthognathic surgery, the orthodontic adagio is always decompensation. In fact, the dentition should ideally follow the skeletal flaws, to correct the arches concomitantly with the bony fragments, which carry the dentition. This leads to projected open bites or overclosures in preparing the arches for significant asymmetries in orthognathic surgery. Mutual information and coordination of orthodontist and surgeon are of paramount importance in designing a treatment plan for asymmetric patients.
2. Asymmetric paranasal fullness may be addressed to some extent by paranasal bone reduction; this trick is of limited value due to the root of the canine which needs to be left undisturbed. Paranasal filling with fat transfer or semi-permanent fillers may be helpful to augment the concave site. Mostly, filling techniques should be postponed to a secondary stage instead of during orthognathic surgery.[20]
3. In midface asymmetries, underprojection or overprojection of the zygoma prominence may be addressed by a unilateral transoral zygoma sandwich osteotomy. This will increase the zygomatic projection in both lateral and anterior direction.[21]
4. Asymmetries in the shape of the maxillary arch are difficult to treat. A surgically assisted rapid maxillary expansion is to consider in the initial phases of the treatment, but at that point, it is easily overlooked and causes problems later in achieving maximal occlusion.
5. In cases with unilateral condylar hyperactivity as in UCH, a condylectomy is indicated. Preoperative virtual planning may be used to resect a vertically larger segment of the condyle to instantly reduce the condyle/ramus length, toward more mandibular symmetry.[22]

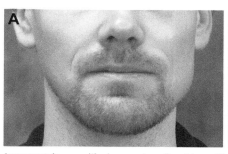
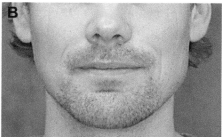

Fig. 8. (*A*) Asymmetric mandibular angles after bimaxillary orthognathic surgery due to flaring of the left angle and inversion of the right angle because of a yaw-correction. (*B*) Contour correction of the mandibular angles with a small reduction (ostectomy) on the left side and an augmentation with a patient-specific PEEK implant on the right side.

6. In cases of unilateral mandibular hypoplasia, such as in craniofacial microsomia or postankylosis hypoplasia in children, ramus elongation may be achieved with distraction osteogenesis or uncommon osteotomies, such as an inverted-L osteotomy.[23]

7. Virtual orthognathic planning will influence choices on chin positioning and mandibular contouring. Virtual planning of the chin position is very well possible in virtual planning software and may be converted with either traditional crafts or patient-specific cutting and drilling guides and patient-specific osteosynthesis material[24] (**Fig. 7**).

8. Mandibular border and angle contouring are more difficult to plan virtually, as condylar rotations and seating are hard to predict in 3D virtual planning and may, therefore, be postponed to second stage virtual planning and surgery. Reduction techniques, such as lower border and mandibular angle osteotomies, or augmentation techniques, such as alloplastic implants and patient-specific implants, are

preferably planned after the orthognathic results have settled and 3D virtual softtissue planning prediction is possible[25] (**Fig. 8**).

9. In vertical asymmetry of the posterior lower border and angle of the mandible, a roll of the maxillomandibular complex with a bilateral sagittal split osteotomy (BSSO) will *not* result in a correction of the mandibular angle (**Fig. 9**A). With the use of an oblique intraoral vertical ramus osteotomy, the mandibular angle will be part of the distal segment and rotate along with the dentition, chin, and lower border and may nicely correct the vertical dystopia of the angles (**Fig. 9**B).

10. To prevent flaring of a mandibular angle in asymmetric BSSOs with a yaw correction of the distal segment, a lingual split offers great opportunities to align both segments well without flaring of the angle. During virtual orthognathic planning, this problem may be identified already and a lingual split may be incorporated in the surgical plan[26] (**Fig. 10**).

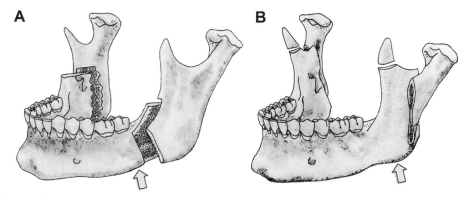

Fig. 9. (*A*) Sagittal split technique; the mandibular angle does not follow the roll in bimaxillary surgery. The arrow points out the rotating distal segment, leaving the mandibular angle as is. (*B*) Intraoral vertical ramus osteotomy; conversely, the mandibular angle does follow the canting movement in bimaxillary surgery with a roll. The arrow shows the mandibular angle that rotates upward as part of the distal segment. (*Courtesy of* R.B. Greebe, DDS.DDS,PhD, Oranjewoud, The Netherlands.)

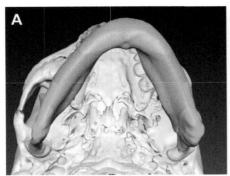
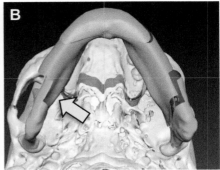

Fig. 10. Worm's-eye view in 3D virtual planning; (*A*) preoperative situation, (*B*) planned situation. The bimaxillary complex is virtually repositioned with a yaw-correction; posterior dentition is rotated toward the right side (*arrow*), an overlap between the anterior and posterior segment in BSSO indicated as a substantial risk for unwanted flaring and jeopardize condylar seating, an additional lingual split on that side may be suitable for the prevention of both.

11. If the mandibular dental arch is asymmetric and unilateral too wide causing transversal problems, such as a cross-bite, a median split may be added to the BSSO to be able to push in a hemimandible for occlusal stability and esthetic purposes.

12. Lower border vertical reduction may be indicated in the substantial vertical asymmetry of the mandibular border. Incidentally, this technique may be hampered by the presence of the infra-alveolar nerve near the lower border. Nerve dissection out of the mandibular canal with a piezotome may be indicated before the ostectomy of the lower border.

CLINICS CARE POINTS

- In midface asymmetries, underprojection or overprojection of the zygoma prominence may be addressed by a unilateral transoral zygoma sandwich osteotomy. This will increase the zygomatic projection in both lateral and anterior direction.

- In cases with unilateral condylar hyperactivity as in UCH, a condylectomy is indicated. Preoperative virtual planning may be used to resect a vertically larger segment of the condyle to instantly reduce the condyle/ramus length, toward more mandibular symmetry.

- To prevent flaring of a mandibular angle in asymmetric BSSOs with a yaw correction of the distal segment, a lingual split offers great opportunities to align both segments well without flaring of the angle. During virtual orthognathic planning, this problem may be identified already and a lingual split may be incorporated in the surgical plan.

REFERENCES

1. Zheng R, Ren D, Xie C, et al. Normality mediates the effect of symmetry on facial attractiveness. Acta Psychol (Amst) 2021;217:103311.
2. Lu SM, Bartlett SP. On facial asymmetry and self-perception. Plast Reconstr Surg 2014;133(6):873e–81e.
3. Wang TT, Wessels L, Hussain G, et al. Discriminative Thresholds in Facial Asymmetry: A Review of the Literature. Aesthet Surg J 2017;37(4):375–85.
4. Lee KH, Kang JW, Lee HY, et al. Ideal Reference Lines for Assessment of Facial Asymmetry in Rhinoplasty Patients. Aesthet Plast Surg 2021. https://doi.org/10.1007/s00266-021-02565-0.
5. Peng L, Cooke MS. Fifteen-year reproducibility of natural head posture: A longitudinal study. Am J Orthod Dentofacial Orthop 1999;116(1):82–5.
6. Kim JY, Kang MH, You JY, et al. Natural Head Postures of Patients With Facial Asymmetry in Frontal View Are Corrected After Orthognathic Surgeries. J Oral Maxillofac Surg 2016;74(2):392–8.
7. Razukevicius SGCSOCD. A "Forced Symmetry": Surgical Planning Protocol for the Treatment of Posterior Facial Asymmetries. EJCO 2016;4:53–9.
8. Djordjevic J, Pirttiniemi P, Harila V, et al. Three-dimensional longitudinal assessment of facial symmetry in adolescents. Eur J Orthod 2013;35(2):143–51.
9. Patel A, Islam SM, Murray K, et al. Facial asymmetry assessment in adults using three-dimensional surface imaging. Prog Orthod 2015;16:36.
10. Lum V, Goonewardene MS, Mian A, et al. Three-dimensional assessment of facial asymmetry using dense correspondence, symmetry, and midline analysis. Am J Orthod Dentofacial Orthop 2020;158(1):134–46.
11. Verhoeven T, Xi T, Schreurs R, et al. Quantification of facial asymmetry: A comparative study of landmark-

based and surface-based registrations. J Craniomaxillofac Surg 2016;44(9):1131–6.

12. Masuoka N, Momoi Y, Ariji Y, et al. Can Cephalometric Indices and Subjective Evaluation Be Consistent for Facial Asymmetry? Angle Orthodontist 2005; 75(4):651–5.

13. Nolte JW, Verhoeven TJ, Schreurs R, et al. 3-Dimensional CBCT analysis of mandibular asymmetry in unilateral condylar hyperplasia. J Craniomaxillofac Surg 2016;44(12):1970–6.

14. Patcas R, Bernini DAJ, Volokitin A, et al. Applying artificial intelligence to assess the impact of orthognathic treatment on facial attractiveness and estimated age. Int J Oral Maxillofac Surg 2019;48(1): 77–83.

15. Bouletreau P, Makaremi M, Ibrahim B, et al. Artificial Intelligence: Applications in orthognathic surgery. J Stomatol Oral Maxillofac Surg 2019;120(4): 347–54.

16. Dot G, Rafflenbeul F, Arbotto M, et al. Accuracy and reliability of automatic three-dimensional cephalometric landmarking. Int J Oral Maxillofac Surg 2020. https://doi.org/10.1016/j.ijom.2020.02.015.

17. Knoops PGM, Papaioannou A, Borghi A, et al. A machine learning framework for automated diagnosis and computer-assisted planning in plastic and reconstructive surgery. Sci Rep 2019;9(1). https://doi.org/10.1038/s41598-019-49506-1.

18. Yurdakurban E, Duran GS, Gorgulu S. Evaluation of an automated approach for facial midline detection and asymmetry assessment: A preliminary study. Orthod Craniofac Res 2021;24(Suppl 2):84–91.

19. Hidaka T, Kurita M, Ogawa K, et al. Application of Artificial Intelligence for Real-Time Facial Asymmetry Analysis. Plast Reconstr Surg 2020;146(2):243e–5e.

20. Lindenblatt N, van Hulle A, Verpaele AM, et al. The Role of Microfat Grafting in Facial Contouring. Aesthet Surg J 2015;35(7):763–71.

21. Mommaerts MY, Abeloos JVS, De Clercq CAS, et al. The 'sandwich' zygomatic osteotomy: technique, indications and clinical results. J Craniomaxillofac Surg 1995;23(1):12–9.

22. Haas Junior OL, Farina R, Hernandez-Alfaro F, et al. Minimally invasive intraoral proportional condylectomy with a three-dimensional printed cutting guide. Int J Oral Maxillofac Surg 2020;49(11): 1435–8.

23. Greaney L, Bhamrah G, Sneddon K, et al. Reinventing the wheel: a modern perspective on the bilateral inverted 'L' osteotomy. Int J Oral Maxillofac Surg 2015;44(11):1325–9.

24. Hany HED, Zaki AH, El Hadidi YN, et al. The Use of Computer-Guided Half Propeller Genioplasty for the Correction of Mandibular Asymmetry (A Mandibular Orthognathic Surgery Without a Condylar Intervention Technical Strategy). J Craniofac Surg 2021. https://doi.org/10.1097/SCS.0000000000008431.

25. Olate S, Huetequeo-Molina C, Requena R, et al. Patient Specific Implants to Solve Structural Facial Asymmetry After Orthognathic Surgery. J Craniofac Surg 2021;32(3):e269–71.

26. Ellis E 3rd. A method to passively align the sagittal ramus osteotomy segments. J Oral Maxillofac Surg 2007;65(10):2125–30.

Management of Bimaxillary Protrusion

Rama Krsna Rajandram, MBBS, DDS, MFDS, MDS-OMFS (HKU), Associate Professor[a],*,
Lavanyah Ponnuthurai, DDS, MClinDent in Prosthodontics (London)[b],
Komalam Mugunam, BDS, MJDF[a], Yunn Shy Chan, BDS, MJDF[a]

KEYWORDS

- Bimaxillary protrusion • Extraction orthodontics • Non-extraction orthodontics
- Obstructive sleep apnea • Orthognathic surgery • Skeletal surgery

KEY POINTS

- All cases of bimaxillary protrusion should be analyzed in holistic manner which includes a subjective and objective assessment.
- Bimaxillary protrusion patients with an underlying Class II skeletal pattern and a hypoplastic chin should receive a full airway assessment to ensure that there is no increased risk to develop obstructive sleep apnea with the orthodontic only approach.
- Treatment planning must be individualized based on each patient's facial type to ensure favorable posttreatment changes in the vertical direction.
- Clinicians should be able to predict the long-term esthetic and functional outcomes and provide a good informed consent especially in patients who receive orthodontics with extractions before skeletal maturity.
- All moderate to severe bimaxillary protrusion cases would benefit from a combined discussion between the oral and maxillofacial surgeon and orthodontist before coming up with a final treatment plan.

INTRODUCTION

Bimaxillary protrusion is a dentofacial deformity trait that can present in all different skeletal patterns. Clinically, the trait is associated with the presence of a protrusive anterior dentoalveolar segment of the maxilla and mandible. This produces an appearance of unsightly protruding anterior teeth, increased procumbence of the lips and a convex lateral facial profile. These clinical features are often perceived negatively with regard to facial attractiveness.[1–6] It can occurs in almost every ethnic group but relatively more common in the Asian and African populations[2,3,7–11]

Patients with this trait often seek esthetic improvements. This is because the clinical features have been shown to lead to negative psychosocial effects translating from poor self-esteem.[1,3,7,10,12–15] The key factor in ensuring good treatment outcome is often focused on ensuring esthetic satisfaction. It is therefore important that the selected treatment modality is able to address the patient's esthetic concern in short term as well as long term.[1,3]

However, very often clinicians find themselves in a dilemma in selecting the right treatment modality. This is due to the heterogeneity of clinical presentation in every patient with bimaxillary protrusion. Bimaxillary protrusion can be treated orthodontically or by a combination of orthodontics with segmental orthognathic surgery. The traditional orthodontic approach to this skeletal trait is often via extractions of all four first premolars to reduce the anterior proclination.

[a] Department of Oral & Maxillofacial Surgery, Faculty of Dentistry, National University of Malaysia, Jalan Raja Muda Abdul Aziz, Kuala Lumpur 50300, Malaysia; [b] Department of Restorative, Faculty of Dentistry, National University of Malaysia, Kuala Lumpur 50300, Malaysia
* Corresponding author.
E-mail addresses: ramakrsna@ppukm.ukm.edu.my (R.K.R.); lavanyah.p@ukm.edu.my (L.P.)

Oral Maxillofacial Surg Clin N Am 35 (2023) 23–35
https://doi.org/10.1016/j.coms.2022.06.006
1042-3699/23/© 2022 Elsevier Inc. All rights reserved.

Advancements related to the usage of skeletal anchorage devices (SADs) in orthodontics have introduced approaches that distalize the anterior segment using a non-extraction protocol. Last, management can include a combined orthodontic and surgical approach which would involve segmental orthognathic surgery.

Treatment planning that focuses on only the biomechanics to correct the anterior proclination without proper clinical analysis can lead to a satisfactory occlusion from a clinical point of view but an unhappy patient from an esthetic point of view. **Fig. 1** is an example of an end point of a case with bimaxillary protrusion. She was treated orthodontically by retraction of the anterior segment with extraction of all four first premolars. The patient however was dissatisfied at the end of the treatment with the esthetic outcome. It is therefore fundamental to have a good approach in reaching a diagnosis that then guides an individualized patient-specific treatment modality.

APPROACH TO DIAGNOSIS

Clinical diagnosis before deciding on the treatment modality of choice depends on the following:

A. Subjective assessment
B. Objective clinical assessment (**Fig. 2**)
C. Radiographic Assessment

Subjective Assessment

Patient factor
Every patient comes with a certain perception of their problem and an expectation on the treatment outcome. They also have an expected timeline for treatment completion. This must be clearly identified at the pretreatment consultation stage. Clinicians must ensure that each patient is aware of the limitations and risks for each treatment approach. An important factor is the age of the patient at the consultation. Identifying growing

patients that should postpone definitive treatment until skeletal maturity is fundamental especially when segmental orthognathic surgery is indicated. **Fig. 1** shows a patient whom received orthodontic treatment at the age of 15 with all four first premolar extractions. She is now 30 years old and dissatisfied with the current aesthetic outcome. Corrective surgery at this point is more complicated because of the previous treatment that included extractions. This highlights the importance of age at the point of consultation. The clinician must be able to ensure a treatment modality that has a good functional and esthetic outcome on skeletal maturity. This is especially important if the treatment involves irreversible interventions such as extractions. The decision of not considering a combined surgical orthodontic approach in an indicated case may lead to compromised outcomes and possible medicolegal implications. Clinicians need to balance patient expectations together with objective clinical findings when coming up with their final treatment plan.

Objective Clinical Assessment

Facial esthetics assessment
Pretreatment facial esthetic assessment guides the initial consultation. It improves patient understanding with regards to the expected posttreatment changes based on the treatment offered. This is especially important in the skeletal immature patients. This assessment can prevent unnecessary extractions that may compromise long-term management of the esthetic component as seen in the case shown in **Fig. 1**.

Facial esthetic assessment involves a frontal and lateral facial analysis. The frontal facial analysis classifies the facial types into mesofacial, brachyfacial, or dolichofacial. This is to ensure posttreatment facial harmony. The pretreatment amount of incisor show at rest is the next important assessment. Retractions of the anterior segment to correct the protrusion can lead to

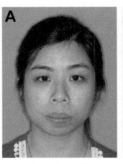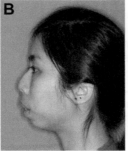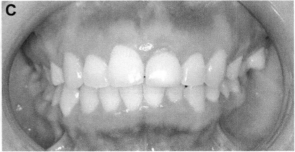

Fig. 1. A patient that came dissatisfied with her posttreatment facial profile and aesthethics. Patient was treated by orthodontics with extractionn before skeletal maturity.

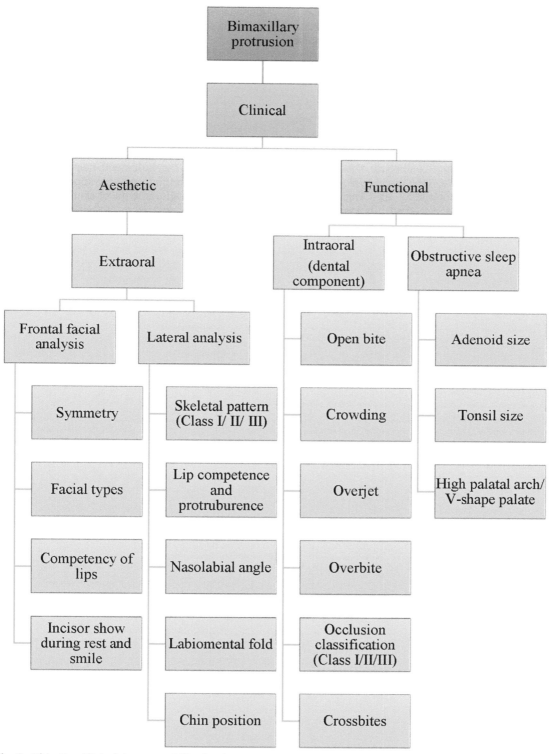

Fig. 2. Objective Clinical Assessment Checkpoints.

changes to the incisal show and upper lip length. These changes should meet the patient's expectations as it has implications to the patient's smile. Underlying concomitant skeletal asymmetries need to be diagnosed to ensure that the patient understands the limitations of each treatment modality in addressing the skeletal asymmetry.

The lateral facial analysis helps to group patients with bimaxillary protrusion to the skeletal Classes I–III. It also identifies a hypoplastic chin. Several soft tissue angles and characteristics play an important role in facial esthetics. These include the nasolabial angle, labiomental fold, and the presence of an incompetent lip. Clinicians must be familiar with the expected changes that will happen to these parameters with each suggested treatment modality.

FUNCTIONAL ASSESSMENT

The presence of functional issues also plays a part in deciding the treatment of choice. Functional assessment includes an airway and dental examination. Airway assessment is important as orthodontic correction of the anterior dentoalveolar proclination by extractions of all four first premolars in the presence of an underlying skeletal Class II, and hypoplastic chin will increase the risk of developing obstructive sleep apnea (OSA) in a susceptible patient. The airway assessment should include tonsil grading, the body mass index, and the presence of transverse discrepancies of the maxilla or a V-shaped maxilla. These are all independent risk factors for OSA. If these factors are present in a patient whom receives extractions for distalization of the anterior segment, the risk for OSA will be potentiated. This group of patients stands to benefit skeletal segmental orthognathic surgery to correct the bimaxillary protrusion as well as to improve their airway parameters.

Next is the dental assessment. This includes identifying space restrictions/crowding, presence of a favorable overjet and overbite, and the angle's classification. These findings lead to the possible need for extractions as well as if SADs or segmental orthognathic should be considered.

RADIOGRAPHIC ASSESSMENT
Lateral Cephalometry

Lateral cephalometry acts as an adjunct to clinical assessment (**Fig. 3**). It provides angular measurements to supplement the diagnosis with regards to skeletal analysis, baseline dental deviations, and esthetic prediction. This enhances the ability of clinicians to give valid information to their patients based on the suggested treatment modality and manage expectations with regards to treatment time and esthetic outcomes.

Lateral cephalometry analysis can be systematically divided to :

- Skeletal Analysis
- Dental Angular Measurements
- Esthetic Predictions

Skeletal Analysis

Skeletal angular measurements help to predict the feasibility of an orthodontic only approach. It gives a prediction on the amount of dental movement that will be needed to correct the bimaxillary protrusion and diagnose any underlying skeletal deformities. It also allows analysis of the posterior pharyngeal space to identify patients at risk of developing OSA posttreatment. The important baselines angles include:

- Sella to Nasion and A-point (SNA): Assessment of the anterior posterior position of the maxilla to indicate if the maxilla is normal, prognathic, or retrognathic.
- Sella to Nasion and B-point (SNB): Assessment of the anterior posterior position of the mandible to determine if the mandible is normal, prognathic, or retrognathic.
- A-point to Nasion and B-point (ANB): This angle will determine if the patient is a skeletal Class I, II, or III.
- Frankfurt-mandibular plane angle (FMPA): This angle will determine the facial proportion and vertical growth pattern of the patient. This helps support the earlier clinical assessment of facial type. This component has an important correlation to the types of biomechanics that need to be considered when correcting the anterior proclination which has an impact to the vertical height of the face. This change must be in favorable to the baseline facial type of the patient.

• Dental angular measurements
This measurement indicates the amount of retraction needed at the level of the anterior incisors to correct the convex lateral facial appearance. This amount indirectly translates to the distal space needed to retract the anterior segment and if this can be achieved by premolar extractions or by the use of skeletal anchorage devices (SADs). In the presence of severe skeletal deformities and discrepancy, the retraction of the anterior segment will require segmental orthognathic surgery.

The important parameters that will need measurement include:

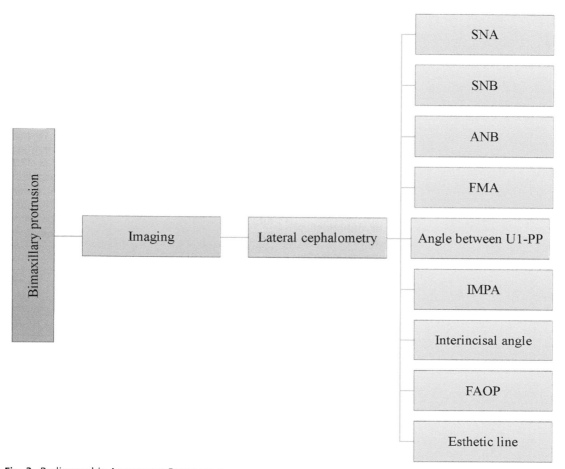

Fig. 3. Radiographic Assessment Parameters.

- Upper incisor to palatal plane (U1-PP): This documents the degree of proclination of the anterior upper incisors.
- Lower incisor mandibular plane angle (IMPA): This documents the degree of proclination of the lower incisors.
- Interincisal angle (IIA): This angle determines the severity of bimaxillary protrusion leading to the procumbence of the incisors.

• *Esthetic predictions*
Functional esthetic occlusal plane The functional esthetic occlusal plane (FAOP) provides important information concerning the (i) vertical relationship of the incisors with the lips at rest and (ii) the position of molars in contact. This facilitates understanding with regards to the limitation of a selected treatment modality to the esthetic and functional demands (occlusion) of the patient. It also provides valuable esthetic information as it analyzes the relationship of the incisor with the lips. This will then indicate if the exposure is within the

acceptable limits according to age. At the same time, it also indicates the reference position of molars and their respective vertical dimension. This assessment is important as it takes into consideration the posttreatment outcome in patients with different skeletal patterns. Bimaxillary protrusion patients stand to benefit significantly from this assessment as it incorporates esthetic outcomes instead of focusing purely on the biomechanics required to correct the angular measurements.

Esthetic plane The esthetic plane (E-plane) is a simple linear line drawn from the tip of the nose to the tip of the chin. It allows for an assessment of the position of the upper lip and lower lip in relation to this line. It has been documented that a pleasant smile is produced if the lower lip is 2 mm behind this line and the upper lip is 4 mm behind this line. This assessment helps the clinician to decide if an extraction protocol or a nonextraction protocol would produce a good smile at the end of the treatment. This line can also determine the degree of concavity or convexity from an underlying skeletal problem that may indirectly indicate the need for segmental orthognathic surgery.

THERAPEUTIC OPTIONS

This review article attempts to group bimaxillary protrusion patients into mild, moderate, and severe. This will improve the ability to screen patients holistically. The grouping suggested is based on the specific clinical and radiographic criteria as shown in **Tables 1** , **2** and **3**. The management suggested for each group is based on the treatment approaches reported in the literature. It can either be via orthodontics only or orthodontics with segmental orthognathic surgery.

The orthodontics only management includes two major approaches. It can either involve orthodontics with all four first premolar/bicuspid extractions or non-extraction orthodontics with intra-alveolar skeletal anchorages devices (SADs). In the latter, the device is used to torque and distalize the anterior segment.

Segmental orthognathic surgery incorporates anterior maxillary segmentalization (Le Fort I segmentalization or Wassmund osteotomy) surgery together with anterior mandibular subapical osteotomies (Hofer/Kole osteotomy) to correct the bimaxillary protrusion. The maxillary anterior segmental osteotomy is done together with the maxillary Le Fort I and bilateral sagittal split osteotomies with the movements dependent on the overall clinical diagnosis of the skeletal deformity. This surgery is technically difficult as the surgical movement requires manipulation at the region of the posterior maxilla to allow the set back of the maxilla. This anatomic area is known to have significant surgical morbidity due to vascular and neurologic risk. The need for segmentalization increases the risk of avascular osteonecrosis and can compromise periodontal health.

Based on the suggested grouping, the authors recommend that mild cases be treated orthodontically. Severe cases should be managed by combined orthodontics and segmental orthognathic surgery. The moderate group, however, is a unique group with regards to management. These cases can be approached orthodontically or by a combination of orthodontics with segmental orthognathic surgery. The decision depends on the patient expectations and the clinicians experience in ensuring that the selected treatment modality can address the patient's expectation. If the patient chooses against segmental orthognathic surgery due to the fear of surgical risk, proper documentation and informed consent

must be taken to ensure that the patient agrees to accept a compromised outcome.

DISCUSSION

Patients with bimaxillary protrusion often seek for esthetic improvement due to the clinical presentation of this trait.[16–19] It is a unique dentofacial deformity trait as very often there is a need to look beyond biomechanics in deciding the treatment approach. The principle behind a nonsurgical orthodontic approach versus a combined orthodontics with segmental orthognathic surgery defers from each other. Orthodontics uprights and retracts the anterior dentition, whereas surgery repositions the anterior segments of the bony jaw. A combined skeletal segmental orthognathic surgery approach

Table 1
Mild bimaxillary protrusion

Treatment Approach: Orthodontics	
Non-Extraction Orthodontics	**Extraction Orthodontics**
Frontal facial assessment: • Competent lips • 1–2 mm incisal show • No skeletal asymmetry • Facial proportion in harmony Lateral facial assessment: • Acute nasolabial angle • Normal to slight changes of labiomental fold Intraoral assessment: • No open bite • Mild overjet and overbite • Class 1 molar occlusion • No crossbites	Frontal facial assessment: • Competent lips • 1–2 mm incisal show • No skeletal asymmetry • Facial proportion in harmony Lateral facial assessment: • Acute nasolabial angle • Shallow labiomental fold Intraoral assessment: • No open bite • Significant over jet and overbite • Class I/II molar occlusion • Presence of crowding
Lateral Cephalometry	
• FAOP increase • U1-PP increase • IMPA increase • IIA decreased (closer to 115.3°) • Horizontal line of lips to E-line increase	• FAOP increase • U1-PP increase • IMPA increase • IIA decreased (closer to 115.3°) • Horizontal line of lips to E-line increase

Table 2
Moderate bimaxillary protrusion

Treatment Approach : Orthodontics OR Combined Orthodontics with Segmental Orthognathic Surgery

Non-Extraction Orthodontics	Extraction Orthodontics	Combined Skeletal Surgery and Orthodontics

Frontal facial assessment:
• Incompetent lips
• No asymmetry
• 1–4 mm incisal show at rest
Lateral facial assessment:
• Acute nasolabial angle
• Obtuse labiomental fold
Intraoral assessment:
• No open bite
• Mild overjet and overbite values
• Class 1 M occlusion
• No crossbites
• Mild crowding
	Frontal facial assessment:
	• Incompetent lips
	• No asymmetry
	• 1–4 mm incisal show at rest
	Lateral facial assessment:
	• Acute nasolabial fold
	• Obtuse labiomental fold
	Intraoral assessment:
	• No open bite
	• Significant over jet and overbite
	• Classes I–III molar occlusion
	• Presence of significant crowding
		Frontal facial assessment:
		• Incompetent lips
		  •Gummy smile with
		    •>4 mm incisal show at rest
		• Presence of any asymmetry/ canting
		Lateral facial assessment:
		• Acute nasolabial angle
		• Obtuse labiomental fold
		Intraoral assessment:
		• Open bite—limit < 3
		• Significant over jet and overbite
		• Classes I–III molar occlusion
		Airway assessment
		• Risk of sleep disordered breathing or OLA

Lateral Cephalometry		
• Skeletal Class 1 • FAOP increased • U1-PP increased • IMPA increase • IIA decreased (significantly reduced from 125°) • Lips less than 2–3 mm protrusive from E-line	• Skeletal Class I and mild skeletal Class II • FAOP increase • U1-PP increase • IMPA increase • IIA decreased (significantly reduced from 125°) • Lips more than 2–3 mm protrusive from E-line	• Significant underlying anterior posterior skeletal discrepancy • Vertical maxillary excess • Hyperdivergent face • FAOP increase • U1-PP increase • IMPA increase • IIA decreased (significantly further from 125°) • Lips more than 2-3 mm protrusive from E-line

can offer a correction that improves the facial profile and balance concurrently with the bimaxillary protrusion. This is especially relevant in the moderate and severe cases.[11] The amount of treatment time as well as the role of orthodontics also differs between these two approaches. The combined orthodontics and segmental orthognathic surgery approach also has more systemic risk which may be a deterring factor to many patients.

Mild Bimaxillary Protrusion

Mild bimaxillary protrusion cases can be managed by orthodontics only (see **Table 1**). This group of patients often presents with an underlying skeletal Class I relationship with minimal deranged soft tissue esthetic parameters. The clinical dilemma in this group of patients often surrounds the need for four premolar/bicuspid extractions. Extraction simplifies and accelerates the ability to correct the dentoalveolar protrusions which is achieved

by closing the extraction space. Cases ideal for non-extraction orthodontics include the absence of crossbites, crowding, and a Class I molar relationship.[20] These cases can incorporate the use of SADs.[21] Types of skeletal anchorage devices reported in the literature with regards to a non-extraction approach to bimaxillary protrusion include intra-alveolar and extra-alveolar screws.[22] A prerequisite to this non-extraction protocol with the SADs is there must be adequate space at the retromolar region. This is to allow distalization of the whole arch.[22] However, there is certain risk associated with this non-extraction approach with mini anchorage screws. The risk includes risk of damage to the adjacent roots due to the limited space available to guide the biomechanics. This increases treatment time.[23] Considerable clinical experience is also needed as there is a need to constantly review and change the mechanics of the force to direct the distalization of

Table 3
Severe bimaxillary protrusion

Combined Segmentalization Orthognathic Surgery and Orthodontics	Lateral Cephalometry
Frontal facial assessment: • Incompetent lips • Gummy smile • Greater than 4 mm incisal show • Presence of any asymmetry/canting Lateral facial assessment: • Acute nasolabial angle • Obtused labiomental fold Intraoral assessment: • Anterior open bite >4 mm • Significant overjet and overbite • Class II/III molar occlusion Airway assessment • Risk of sleep-disordered breathing or obstructive sleep apnea	• Severe anterior-posterior skeletal discrepancies • Vertical maxillary excess • FAOP significantly increased • U1-PP increased • IMPA increased • IIA decreased (significant further from 125°) • Horizontal line of lips to E-line increased

the anterior segment. Patients must therefore be compliant to the need for multiple visits and a longer treatment duration.

Extraction of premolars offers benefits of improvements to the soft tissue esthetics which include the nasolabial and labiomental fold together with correction of the overjet, overbite, and crowding. In cases of a Class II molar relationship, a camouflage effect can be obtained with the extraction of the premolars, thus reducing the procumbence of the lips by 3.4 mm and 3.6 mm in upper and lower lips.[24] **Fig. 4** shows an example of a mild case classified based on the objective clinical assessment mentioned in this article.

Moderate Bimaxillary Protrusion

This group of patients can be managed either by nonsurgical orthodontics or by combined orthodontics with segmental orthognathic surgery (see **Table 2**). Very often patients with a skeletal Class II malocclusion are seen in this group. Important consideration for treatment of choice is based on the amount of soft tissue and skeletal improvement needed as well as the length of treatment time.[20] In moderate cases, patients with incompetent lips, with a 1 to 4 mm incisal show at rest and no other significant skeletal and occlusal derangement as mention in **Table 2** can undergo orthodontic treatment alone.[25] The decision to consider premolars extractions in this group of patients are dependent on the relationship of the lips protrusion to the E-line. Premolar extractions in the nonsurgical orthodontic patient can also camouflage a mild Class II skeletal discrepancy in the

presence of crowding and any significant overjet. The non-extraction methods can be considered if the baseline dental malocclusion (overjet, overbite, molar relationship) is minimal and patients' expectation with regard to esthetics is low. Facial convexity can also be improved with the extractions of the first premolars. It has been shown that the facial convexity reduces an extra 2 to 3 mm in protrusion in comparison to non-extraction cases.[26,27]

Combined segmental orthognathic surgery and orthodontics should be considered if there is any significant asymmetry or vertical skeletal disproportions in addition to all the clinical and radiographic criteria for this group. Vertical skeletal disproportions can be corrected by impaction using the Le Fort I osteotomy which is combined with an anterior segmentalization to improve the bimaxillary protrusion. Patients with radiographically thin anterior alveolar bone are also suitable for surgical cases. This is to avoid any bony dehiscence or root resorption due to the need for retraction forces.[20,28]

Fig. 5 shows the importance of the age of the patient in deciding the treatment modality of choice in patients grouped as moderate bimaxillary protrusion. Extractions in their growth phase to correct the bimaxillary protrusion may lead to complications related to poor esthetic outcome as well as increased risk of OSA later if they are susceptible. **Fig. 6** shows another case of moderate bimaxillary protrusion based on our criteria which can be treated by orthodontics with extractions.

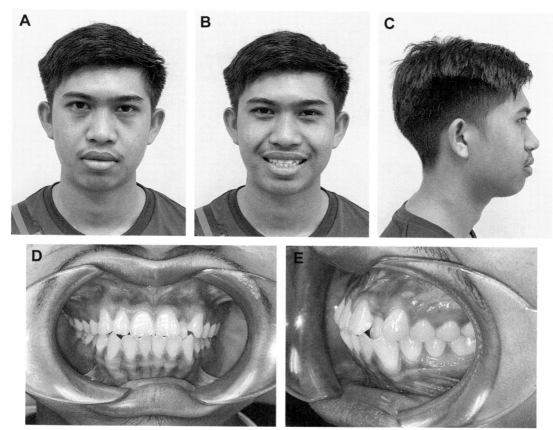

Fig. 4. Mild bimaxillary protrusion.

Severe Bimaxillary Protrusion

These patients have significant underlying skeletal discrepancies (**Table 3**) Combined skeletal segmental orthognathic surgery and orthodontics offers an ideal solution to these patients with regard to functional and esthetics demands as well as long-term stability.[10] Skeletal surgery is able to overcome the periodontal and alveolar housing limitations, extend the achievable range of tooth movement, provide faster retraction rate which in turn leads to a higher rate of space closure with better anchorage control.[2,29–31] This indirectly leads to the reduced treatment time and is suitable for adults who are desirous for shorter treatment time with significant functional and esthetic expectations.[4,8,32] Surgery has an advantage over the conventional nonsurgical orthodontic treatment because it offers simultaneous three-dimensional skeletal correction which includes (i) severe incisor proclination; (ii) extreme anterior open bite and deep bite; and (iii) vertical or antero-posterior discrepancy.[8,30] Surgery also allows for larger basal bone retraction which in turn provides a greater change in upper lip projection compared with orthodontic treatment alone.[2] Thus, instant and optimal effect of esthetic facial results can be obtained from the surgery when compared with orthodontics alone.[4,8,29,33]

Special Consideration Group

Patients with moderate and severe bimaxillary protrusion may also present with risk of sleep-disordered breathing which includes OSA.[34] Risk factors for OSA in patients with bimaxillary protrusion include a Class II facial pattern, brachyfacial type, presence of a small or retruded mandible and chin, elongated face, chronic mouth breathers secondary to the hypertrophy of the inferior turbinate's, enlarged adenoids and tonsils, deep and narrow hard palate, and long soft palate.[35–37] It is especially important to screen all bimaxillary protrusion patients with these clinical features. This is to avoid an only orthodontic approach with extraction of all four first premolars that is often followed by retraction and retroclination of the maxillary and mandibular incisors to close the

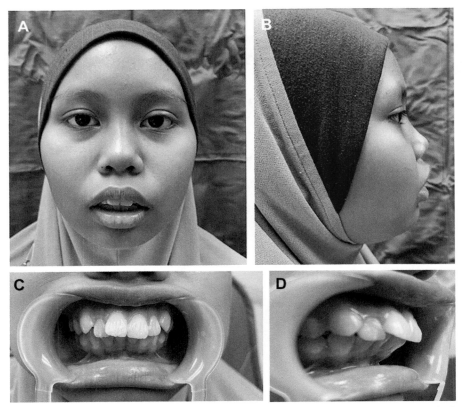

Fig. 5. Growing child with moderate bimaxillary protrusion.A case suitable to avoid extractions before skeletal maturity in view a clincal risk of susceptibility to obstructive sleep apnea (OSA). The case has indications for possible conbined orthodontics with skeletal segmentalization surgery.

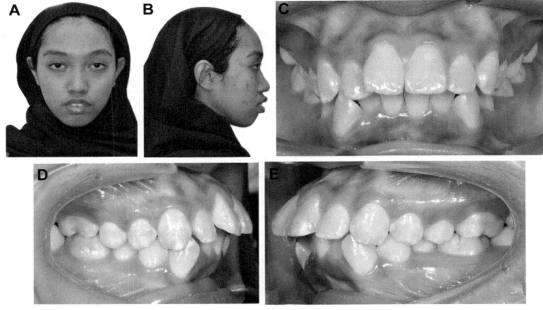

Fig. 6. Moderate bimaxillary protrusion case that can be treated by premolar extractions.

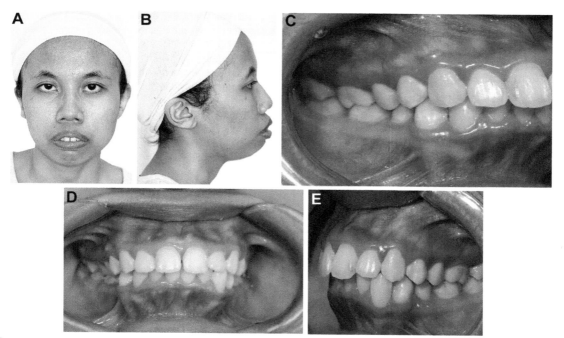

Fig. 7. Severe bimaxillary case.

extraction spaces.[2,3,7,38] This leads to oropharyngeal crowding, which develops secondary to the posterior dislocation of the hyoid bone as the anterior segment is distalized. This then decreases the cross-sectional area behind the soft palate and uvula.[14,38,39] Besides that, the retraction of the incisors leads to a reduction in tongue's space. The tongue may then fall backward and eventually increases the risk of airway obstruction during sleep.[5,14,39] Segmental orthognathic surgery should be considered in individuals with bimaxillary protrusion presenting with risk factors for OSA. Anterior segmental osteotomy of the maxilla offers an added advantage to correction of the anterior proclination. It has been shown to exert a minimal effect on the pharyngeal airway in comparison to orthodontic treatment only.[4] In cases with severe deficiency of the chin, skeletal surgery approach offers the advantage of doing a simultaneous genioplasty to achieve better facial profile as well as increasing posterior airway space.[2] **Fig. 7** shows an example of a case that should receive a combined surgical and orthodontic management as it falls under the severe group and also the special consideration group. She is at risk of developing OSA if she receives only orthodontic treatment with extractions of premolars.

As with all surgeries there are major risks involved in comparison to the nonsurgical orthodontic approach. This should be well communicated to patients before any treatment is started to ensure patients are fully aware and agreeable to proceed with the suggested treatment.

SUMMARY

Approach to the management of bimaxillary protrusion requires clinicians to look beyond biomechanics only. There is a need for a comprehensive approach that ensures long-term esthetic and functional outcomes. Multidisciplinary discussion involving orthodontists and oral and maxillofacial surgeons at the pretreatment stage especially in the moderate and severe cases with functional requirements should be recommended. Failure to individualized treatment planning based on age, esthetics, and functional requirement can lead to the perceived treatment failure by patients in the long term despite a satisfactory occlusion.

CLINICS CARE POINTS

- All patients with bimaxillary protrusion which are from the growing age population with an underlying Class II skeletal profile and requiring premolar extractions should be screened for underlying risk of worsening of oropharyngeal crowding and chronic mouth breathing to avoid risk of progression to obstructive sleep apnea when they are older. This group may benefit multimodal and multidisciplinary management.

- Airway screening prior to orthodontic extractions should include:

  o Identfying underlying presence of nasal obstruction that leads to chronic mouth breathing

  o Anatomic risk factors for oropharyngeal crowding:

    i. Reduced tongue space that includes transverse discrepancy of the maxilla or V-shaped maxilla.

    ii. Severe tongue scalloping that maybe due to constricted tongue space secondary to the presence of mandibular tori or macroglossia.

    iii. Skeletal Class II discrepancy.

    iv. Genio-hypoplasia in anterior posterior.

    v. Adenoid and tonsillar hypertrophy.

    vi. Friedmans (Natural tongue position) Classification. Increased risk if >Class 11.

REFERENCES

1. Chu QS, Schwartz G, de Bono J, et al. Phase I and pharmacokinetic study of lapatinib in combination with capecitabine in patients with advanced solid malignancies. J Clin Oncol 2007;25(24):3753–8.

2. Xie F, Teng L, Jin X, et al. Systematic analysis of clinical outcomes of anterior maxillary and mandibular subapical osteotomy with preoperative modeling in the treatment of bimaxillary protrusion. J Craniofac Surg 2013;24(6):1980–6.

3. Chu Y-M, Bergeron L, Chen Y-R. Bimaxillary Protrusion : An Overview of the Surgical-Orthodontic Treatment. Semin Plast Surg 2009;23(1):32–9. https://doi.org/10.1055/s-0028-1110099.

4. Blankenstein TN, Smith DAJ, Cheng AJL. A linear density on imaging: Non-contrast CT as a useful localisation method. Ann Acad Med Singap 2021;50(8):660–1.

5. Alessandrino F, Smith DA, Spierling A, et al. Cancer Clinical Trials: What Every Radiologist Wants to Know but Is Afraid to Ask. AJR Am J Roentgenol 2021;216(4):1099–111.

6. Downs LO, Vawda S, Bester PA, et al. Bimodal distribution and set point HBV DNA viral loads in chronic infection: retrospective analysis of cohorts from the UK and South Africa. Wellcome Open Res 2020;5:113.

7. Oueis R, Waite PD, Wang J, et al. Orthodontic-Orthognathic Management of a patient with skeletal class II with bimaxillary protrusion, complicated by vertical maxillary excess: A multi-faceted case report of difficult treatment management issues. Int Orthod 2020;18(1):178–90.

8. Ogundipe O, Otuyemi O. Surgical and orthodontic treatment methods in patients with bimaxillary protrusion-a systematic review. J West Afr Coll Surgeons 2017;7(2):31.

9. Ahmad Nasir S, Ramli R, Abd Jabar N. Predictors of enophthalmos among adult patients with pure orbital blowout fractures. PloS one 2018;13(10):e0204946.

10. Chen G, Teng F, Xu T-M. Distalization of the maxillary and mandibular dentitions with miniscrew anchorage in a patient with moderate Class I bimaxillary dentoalveolar protrusion. Am J Orthod Dentofacial Orthop 2016;149(3):401–10.

11. Solem RC, Marasco R, Guiterrez-Pulido L, et al. Three-dimensional soft-tissue and hard-tissue changes in the treatment of bimaxillary protrusion. Am J Orthod Dentofacial Orthop 2013;144(2):218–28.

12. Ramos CJ. Treatment of dental and skeletal bimaxillary protrusion in patient with Angle Class I malocclusion. Dental Press J Orthodontics 2013;18(6):130–7.

13. Liu R, Hou W-B, Yang P-Z, et al. Severe skeletal bimaxillary protrusion treated with micro-implants and a self-made four-curvature torquing auxiliary: A case report. World J Clin cases 2021;9(3):722.

14. Bhatia S, Jayan B, Chopra SS. Effect of retraction of anterior teeth on pharyngeal airway and hyoid bone position in Class I bimaxillary dentoalveolar protrusion. Med J Armed Forces India 2016;72(Suppl 1):S17–23.

15. Alqahtani N, Alshammari R, Almoammar K, et al. Post-orthodontic cephalometric variations in bimaxillary protrusion cases managed by premolar extraction—A retrospective study. Niger J Clin Pract 2019;22(11):1530.

16. Kim J.R., Son W.S., Lee S.G. A retrospective analysis of 20 surgically corrected bimaxillary protrusion patients. Int J Adult Orthodon Orthognath Surg. 17 (1), 2002, 23-7. PMID: 11934052.

17. Tan SK, Leung WK, Tang ATH, et al. Facial profile study using 3-dimensional photographs to assess esthetic preferences of Hong Kong Chinese orthognathic patients and laypersons. Am J Orthod Dentofacial Orthop 2022;161(2):e105–13.

18. Farrow AL, Zarrinnia K, Azizi K. Bimaxillary protrusion in black Americans—an esthetic evaluation and the treatment considerations. Am J Orthod Dentofacial Orthop 1993;104(3):240–50.

19. Huang Y-P, Li W-r. Correlation between objective and subjective evaluation of profile in bimaxillary protrusion patients after orthodontic treatment. Angle Orthodontist 2015;85(4):690–8.

20. Baek S-H, Kim B-H. Determinants of successful treatment of bimaxillary protrusion: orthodontic

treatment versus anterior segmental osteotomy. J Craniofac Surg 2005;16(2):234–46.

21. Kyung H-M. Overview development of orthodontic micro-implants for intraoral anchorage. J Clin Orthod 2003;37:321–8.

22. Villela HM. Treatment of bimaxillary protrusion using intra-and extra-alveolar miniscrews associated to self-ligating brackets system. Dental Press J Orthod 2020;25:66–84.

23. Chung K-R, Choo H, Kim S-H, et al. Timely relocation of mini-implants for uninterrupted full-arch distalization. Am J Orthod Dentofacial Orthop 2010; 138(6):839–49.

24. Drobocky OB, Smith RJ. Changes in facial profile during orthodontic treatment with extraction of four first premolars. Am J Orthod Dentofacial Orthop 1989;95(3):220–30.

25. Keating PJ. The Treatment of Bimaxillary Protrusion: A cephalometric consideration of changes in the inter-incisal angle and soft tissue profile. Br J Orthod 1986;13(4):209–20.

26. Luppanapornlarp S, Johnston LE Jr. The effects of premolar-extraction: a long-term comparison of outcomes in "clear-cut" extraction and nonextraction Class II patients. Angle Orthodontist 1993;63(4): 257–72.

27. Lewis SJ. Bimaxillary Protrusion. Angle Orthodontist 1943;13(3):51–9.

28. Xia K, Wang J, Yu L, et al. Dentofacial characteristics and age in association with incisor bony support in adult female patients with bimaxillary dentoalveolar protrusion. Orthod Craniofac Res 2021;24(4): 585–92.

29. Nielsen AMW, Ojkic D, Dutton CJ, et al. Aquatic bird bornavirus 1 infection in a captive Emu (Dromaius novaehollandiae): presumed natural transmission from free-ranging wild waterfowl. Avian Pathol 2018;47(1):58–62.

30. Gupta A, Sharma SD, Kataria V, et al. Experience with Anterior Maxillary Osteotomy Techniques: A Prospective Study of 20 Cases. J Maxill Oral Surg 2020;19(1):119–24.

31. Sakthi SV, Vikraman B, Shobana V, et al. Corticotomy-assisted retraction: an outcome assessment. Indian J Dental Res 2014;25(6):748.

32. Shimazaki K, Otsubo K, Yonemitsu I, et al. Severe unilateral scissor bite and bimaxillary protrusion treated by horseshoe Le Fort I osteotomy combined with mid-alveolar osteotomy. Angle Orthodontist 2014;84(2):374–9.

33. Bhagat SK, Kannan S, Babu M, et al. Soft Tissue Changes Following Combined Anterior Segmental Bimaxillary Orthognathic Procedures. J Maxillofacial Oral Surg 2019;18(1):93–9.

34. Banabilh S, Samsudin A, Suzina A, et al. Facial profile shape, malocclusion and palatal morphology in Malay obstructive sleep apnea patients. Angle Orthodontist 2010;80(1):37–42.

35. Cohen-Lévy J, Contencin P, Couloigner V. Craniofacial morphology and obstructive sleep apnea: the role of dento-facial orthopedics. J Dentofacial Anom Orthod 2009;12(3):108–20.

36. Anand AM, Bharadwaj R, Krishnaswamy NR. Role of facial pattern in patients with obstructive sleep apnea among the South Indian (Chennai) population: a cross-sectional study. J Dent Sleep Med 2020;7(1).

37. Capistrano A, Cordeiro A, Capelozza Filho L, et al. Facial morphology and obstructive sleep apnea. Dental Press J Orthodontics 2015;20:60–7.

38. Aldosari MA, Alqasir AM, Alqahtani ND, et al. Evaluation of the airway space changes after extraction of four second premolars and orthodontic space closure in adult female patients with bimaxillary protrusion–A retrospective study. Saudi dental J 2020;32(3):142–7.

39. Chen Y, Hong L, Wang CL, et al. Effect of large incisor retraction on upper airway morphology in adult bimaxillary protrusion patients. Angle Orthod 2012;82(6):964–70.

Surgical Management for Vertical Maxillary Excess

Hao Wu, MD[a,b,c],*, Dongming He, MD[a,b,c], Yong Wu, MD[d], Lingyong Jiang, MD, Prof[a,b,c],*, Xudong Wang, MD, Prof[a,b,c],*

KEYWORDS

- Vertical maxillary excess • Orthognathic surgery • Le Fort I osteotomy • Lip–incisor relationship
- Computer-assisted surgical plan • Maxillary impaction

KEY POINTS

- Vertical maxillary excess (VME) is a common maxillofacial deformity affecting the lower third of face, which can take place in posterior, anterior, and total maxilla.
- Orthognathic surgery is the workhorse to correct VME of adult patients via bone removal and maxilla impaction, which can be carried out in posterior, anterior, or total maxilla.
- Preoperative computer-assisted three-dimensional surgical plans show great importance due to the prediction of orthognathic surgery.
- The lower anterior facial height and relationship of upper lip–incisor (ie, the exposure of upper incisor in repose) is critical for the determination of the maxilla repositioning.

INTRODUCTION

Patients with vertical maxillary excess (VME) often show excessive vertical maxillary development, which can take place in the whole, posterior, or anterior maxilla, and thus termed as total VME, posterior VME, and anterior VME, respectively.[1] Sometimes it is also named as long face deformity and the clinical features include long face, gummy smile, and occasionally open bite.[2] Approximately 20%–30% of patients show a vertical increase of the lower third part of the face.[3,4] It is challenging to correct the long face deformity of patients with VME. There seem no better choices for the adult patient than the combination of orthodontic and orthognathic surgery, which consists of preoperative orthodontics, orthognathic surgery, and postoperative orthodontics.[5]

After preoperative orthodontic treatment, orthognathic surgery will be carried out to correct deformities, which has been the workhorse for the management of VME for decades.[6] The Le Fort I osteotomy of the maxilla makes it feasible to impact maxillary dentoalveolus via bone removal. Then, the mandible will autorotate anteriorly around the condylar hinge axis, which was first described in the 1970s.[7,8] On this basis, plenty of surgical techniques have been developed for the management of different kinds of VME. The direction and extent of planned surgical repositioning depend on the original deformity. When planning maxillary impaction, the most significant factors for determination are the low anterior facial height (LAFH) and resultant upper lip–incisor relationship, which is the mainstay of the treatment planning.[1] Furthermore, the application of a computer-assisted three-dimensional (3D) surgical plan can

[a] Department of Oral & Cranio-Maxillofacial Surgery, Shanghai Ninth People's Hospital, College of Stomatology, Shanghai Jiao Tong University School of Medicine, No.639, Zhizaoju Road, Shanghai 200011, PR China; [b] National Clinical Research Center for Oral Diseases, No.639, Zhizaoju Road, Shanghai 200011, PR China; [c] Shanghai Key Laboratory of Stomatology & Shanghai Research Institute of Stomatology, No.639, Zhizaoju Road, Shanghai 200011, PR China; [d] Shanghai Wuyong Dental Clinic, 255 Lanhua Road, Shanghai 201204, China

* Corresponding authors. Department of Oral & Cranio-Maxillofacial Surgery, Shanghai Ninth People's Hospital, No.639, Zhizaoju Road, Shanghai 200011, PR China.
E-mail addresses: wuhao9464@163.com (H.W.); 247416218@qq.com (L.J.); xudongwang70@hotmail.com (X.W.)

Oral Maxillofacial Surg Clin N Am 35 (2023) 37–48
https://doi.org/10.1016/j.coms.2022.06.012
1042-3699/23/© 2022 Elsevier Inc. All rights reserved.

visualize the bone movement during surgery pre-operatively and make the surgical plan more accurate.

This review is focused on surgical approaches for the management of total, anterior, and posterior VME, depending on different clinical features, which will be described in this review. Computer-assisted 3D surgical plan will also be introduced for accurate virtual plan of orthognathic surgery. Based on the ideal upper lip–incisor relationship, the different surgical plan will be put forward for individual patient to impact maxilla and correct deformities. A typical clinical case is presented to demonstrate the surgical management of a patient with VME as a summary.

CLINICAL FEATURES
Mandible Rotation

Patients with VME often show mandibular rotation backward, which will affect the position of sagittal chin prominence and mandibular plane angle (**Fig. 1**). In general, patients' mandibles will rotate backward and downward if they have normal or reduced length, which will make the chin less prominent and increase the mandibular plane angle (**Fig. 2A**). However, if patients have long mandibles, the chin is rotated to a more normal sagittal position (**Fig. 2B**).

Nasal Morphology

Patients with VME tend to show narrow noses with narrow alar bases (**Fig. 3A**). Prominent nasal dorsa can be observed in patients with long face deformity.

Lip Incompetence

Patients with VME often show an incomplete lip seal (≥4 mm) (**Fig. 3B**), resulting from LAFH increase, the lack of upper and lower lip heights, and the backward mandibular rotation. The interlabial distance at rest and the extent of lip incompetence will increase when these deformities are more severe.

Palatal Vault Morphology

Patients with VME often show high and narrow palatal vaults (**Fig. 3C**), which might be caused by the tongue position, as well as compensatory overeruption of the maxillary dentition resulting from the increased LAFH. As a result, patients with VME may also show posterior dental crossbite.

Anterior Open Bite

The primary etiologic factor of anterior open bite is the excessive face height caused by VME and the resultant clockwise rotation of the mandible, which often happens in patients with posterior and total VME (**Fig. 3D**). The degree of anterior open bite is determined by the LAFH, the compensatory overeruption of incisors and the tongue resting position. However, if patients show the clockwise rotation of maxillary occlusal plane, the anterior open bite may not occur generally.

Upper Lip–Incisor Relationship

The upper lip–incisor relation (ie, exposure of maxillary incisors at rest) is determined by the degree of vertical maxillary development of the anterior dentoalveolar. Thus, for patients with total and anterior VME, the exposure of maxillary incisors will increase. However, patients with posterior VME may show impeded anterior dentoalveolar because of the forward resting tongue position, where the maxillary incisor exposure can be normal or even reduced.

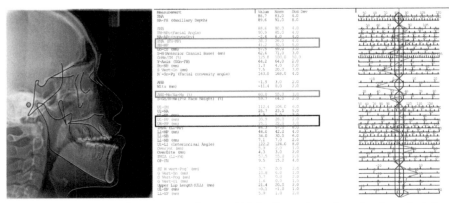

Fig. 1. 2D cephalometric analysis of a patient with a total VME. The red quadrangles show that the mandibular plane angle and LAFH were increased and the mandible was rotated downward. The black quadrangle demonstrates the entirely excess development of the maxilla.

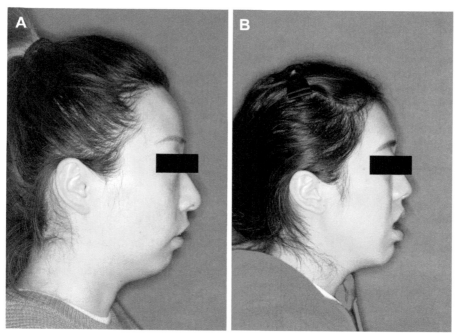

Fig. 2. Patients with VME show backward rotation of the mandible. (*A*) Patient with a short mandible shows a less prominent chin profile. (*B*) The chin of a patient with long mandible is rotated to a more normal sagittal position.

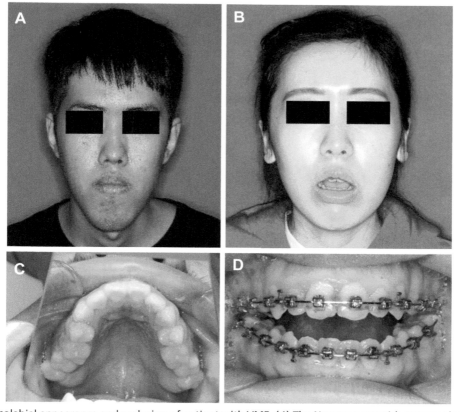

Fig. 3. Nasolabial appearance and occlusion of patient with VME. (*A*) The Narrow nose with narrow alar base. (*B*) An obvious incomplete lip seal. (*C*) The high and narrow palatal vault. (*D*) Anterior open bite.

Gingival Exposure

"Gummy smile" (ie, gingival exposure when smiling) can be observed both anteriorly and posteriorly, which depends on the extent of VME. Patients with total VME often show increased gingival exposure both anteriorly and posteriorly, whereas patients with anterior and posterior VME only show excessive gingival exposure in the overdeveloped regions (**Fig. 4**).

Maxillary Occlusal Plane

The rotation of the maxillary occlusal plane depends on the differences of posterior and anterior vertical excess. Its counterclockwise rotation often results from posterior VME and total VME with excessive posterior maxilla growth. Meanwhile, if the anterior maxilla shows greater vertical excess, a clockwise rotation of the maxillary occlusal plane will appear, including anterior and total VME.

PREOPERATIVE ORTHODONTICS

Generally, the preoperative orthodontic treatments are carried out to prepare for maxillary impaction and subsequent mandibular autorotation. For reduction of the LAFH, the mandibular arch should be leveled as far as possible in the preoperative stage, including incisor intrusion and premolar/molar extrusion. For patients with severe anterior open bite, it is better to align the arch in segments and deviate the roots for the subsequent segmental osteotomy. Furthermore, if a two-piece segmental Le Fort I osteotomy is required to adjust the maxillary dentition transversely, the dental arch should be aligned with the alveolar base.

PREOPERATIVE SURGICAL PLAN
Determining Factors

The orthognathic surgeries for patients with VME generally include maxillary impaction and subsequent counterclockwise mandibular autorotation. When planning the maxillary impaction, the key factors are LAFH and upper lip–incisor relationship, among which the desired exposure of maxillary incisor at rest should be firstly considered. For young adult men, the proper exposure of maxillary incisor at rest is approximately 2 to 3 mm, and about 4 to 5 mm for young adult women. It is also important to plan a slight increase of the maxillary incisor display, considering aging changes of the upper lip. If patients' maxillary incisor exposure is not excessive and a complete lip seal can be achieved, the increase of face height can be acceptable.

Since the final position of mandible and bony chin depends on the movement of maxilla, it is important to avoid excessive impaction to keep balance of the LAFH, total face height, and the standing height of the patient. Furthermore, excessive impaction may cause unwanted changes of the soft tissue, such as elevation of the nasal tip, broadening of the nasal alar base, and a vertically over-compressed "bunched-up" appearance of the midfacial soft tissues.

To mitigate these disadvantages, Rosen[9] suggested undercorrecting in the vertical dimension

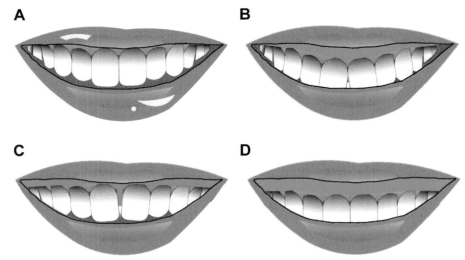

Fig. 4. Schematic of different gingival exposure of smile. (*A*) Normal smile without excessive gingival exposure. (*B*) Excessive anterior gingival exposure. (*C*) Excessive posterior gingival exposure. (*D*) Excessive anterior and posterior gingival exposure.

and overcorrecting in the sagittal dimension. Venkatesh Anehosur and colleagues[10] also reported a modified Le Fort I osteotomy, where the group carried out the osteotomy below the piriform aperture. After follow-up for 1 year, the width of the alar base showed minimal changes, with the width of 36 mm compared with 34 mm preoperatively. The change of soft tissue could be acceptable even though the maxillary impaction was radical.

Besides, other factors should also be considered before orthognathic surgery, such as sagittal and horizontal position of maxilla, transverse width of the dental arches, and correction of the occlusal curve.

Computer-Assisted Surgical Plan

Two-dimensional (2D) cephalometric analysis and model surgery are conventional methods for preoperative surgical plan. However, 2D images could not provide full information about the 3D structures and unexpected problems might occur during surgery, such as bony collision, rotation discrepancy, midline difference and chin inadequacy.[11]

Computer-assisted virtual planning provides a more accurate and predictable approach for orthognathic surgery,[12,13] which integrates surgical plan and intervention via commercial software programs, such as Dolphin Imaging, Maxilim, 3DMDvultus, InVivo-Dental, and SimPlant OMS. 3D diagnostic assessments of facial morphology

can make clinical decisions more precisely, and improve surgical outcomes significantly.[14] The steps of computer-assisted orthognathic surgical plan are listed below (**Fig. 5**):

- Collecting diagnostic data, including clinical examinations, dental models, 3D photographic examinations, MRI, and CT;
- Joint consultation and treatment planning with the orthodontist, surgeon, and the patient;
- Making diagnosis according to a comprehensive analysis of diagnostic data;
- Reconstructing and segmenting anatomic 3D structures in the virtual computer planning;
- Simulating surgical movements and outcomes;
- Designing individualized surgical splints.

SURGICAL MANAGEMENT OF VERTICAL MAXILLARY EXCESS
Surgical Techniques

Le Fort I osteotomy
Le Fort I osteotomy is usually applied for correcting maxillary deformities. Developed by Obwegeser,[15,16] the modern Le Fort I maxillary osteotomy has already been the workhorse for maxilla repositioning, which permits bone removal of maxilla and allows impaction of the maxillary dentoalveolus to achieve ideal occlusion (**Fig. 6**A). It is a relatively safe surgical technique with the complication rate ranging from 4% to 11.7%.[17–19]

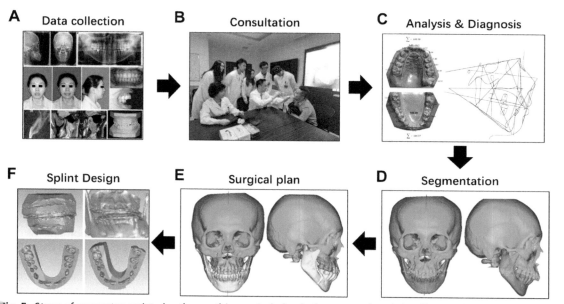

Fig. 5. Steps of computer-assisted orthognathic surgical plan before operation. (*A*) Collecting diagnostic data. (*B*) Joint consultation and treatment planning. (*C*) Data analysis and diagnosis. (*D*) Reconstruction and segmentation. (*E*) Surgical plan and simulation. (*F*) Designing individualized surgical splints.

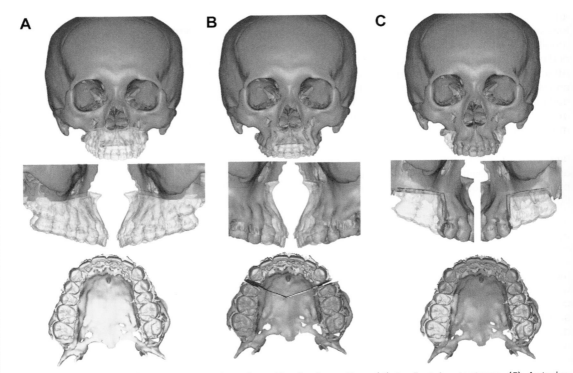

Fig. 6. Schematic of different osteotomies of maxilla for impaction. (*A*) Le Fort I osteotomy. (*B*) Anterior segmental osteotomy. (*C*) Posterior segmental osteotomy.

Anterior segmental osteotomy

The anterior segmental osteotomy was first reported by Wassmund in 1935 to set back the anterior maxillary dentoalveolus.[20] With its development, the anterior segmental osteotomy has been widely used for repositioning of the anterior dentoalveolar segment (**Fig. 6**B). Furthermore, in combination with Le Fort I osteotomy, separate impaction and rotation of anterior and posterior segments can be achieved to create a normal maxillary occlusal plane. Compared with conventional Le Fort I maxilla osteotomy, the anterior segmental osteotomy can determine the postoperative occlusal plane, reduce the risk of relapse and prevent unwanted esthetic changes. A 5-year follow-up research has proved the stability of postoperative occlusion of anterior segmental osteotomy,[21] yet attention should be paid to the postoperative stabilization of the segments.[22]

Posterior segmental osteotomy

Posterior segmental osteotomy of maxilla is an alternative procedure for patients with VME.[23] It is able to reestablish occlusal curves and the vertical position of posterior dentition (**Fig. 6**C), which will improve occlusal relationships with minor surgical injury.[24] Kyung-Hwan Kwon and Sung-Kwon Choi used posterior maxillary segmental osteotomy to treat a 25-year-old male patient with anterior open bite. With the application of skeletal anchorages, the maxillary posterior teeth were impacted up to 3.5 mm and the posterior gingival exposure was improved.[25] It is necessary to a make space for segmental repositioning preoperatively, which largely depends on surgeons' experience and choice, as well as the patient's deformity.

Surgical Treatments

Total vertical maxillary excess

As for patients with total VME, Le Fort I osteotomy is usually applied for maxillary impaction and rotation. It is critical to determine the final position of maxillary incisors, which will help to decide the bone removal of the maxilla.[26] Generally, the amount of bone removal depends on the extent of the excessive vertical development of the maxilla and the rotation of the maxillary occlusal plane. If the patient's maxillary occlusal plane is normal and direct impaction is sufficient to correct the deformity, the amount of anterior and posterior bone removal will be the similar. It is also acceptable to have differential bone removal anteriorly and posteriorly if the maxilla should be rotated to correct the abnormal maxillary occlusal plane, which is also called differential maxillary impaction.[27]

Furthermore, if the desired occlusal curve could not be achieved by preoperative orthodontics, Le Fort I osteotomy can be segmentalized, where segments can be differentially impacted and rotated for the desired dentition alignment. With the help of digital techniques, the maxillary osteotomy and repositioning can be carried out more accurately.[28]

Anterior vertical maxillary excess

As for patients with anterior VME, since the posterior maxilla does not show vertical excess growth, anterior segmental osteotomy can be applied separately to impact the anterior dentoalveolus and to correct "gummy smile."[29] The repositioning of the anterior segment is dependent on the ideal upper lip–incisor relationship as well as the final occlusion. Pre-operatively, the dentition should be aligned in segments and make space for the subsequent osteotomy. Le Fort I osteotomy can also be applied separately or together with an anterior segmental osteotomy, where the maxilla will be rotated counterclockwise to impact anterior dentoalveolaus and to achieve a desired occlusal plane.

Of note, orthodontic treatment can also be an alternative if patients are not willing to accept orthognathic surgery.[30] The key to orthodontic treatment is the intrusion of anterior teeth. In these cases, it is important to control the vertical dimension of the mandibular arch, as the mandibular

teeth tend to extrude spontaneously with the intrusion of maxillary teeth.[31,32] For adult patients, temporary anchorage devices (TADs) have been widely used to perform intrusive retraction of the anterior maxillary teeth to correct gummy smile, which has been reported by many studies.[33–35] However, if patients show severe VME, orthognathic surgery can achieve a more profound result.

Posterior vertical maxillary excess

As for patients with posterior VME, anterior open bite is a common feature due to the clockwise rotation of the mandible. If the upper lip–incisor relationship should be corrected, Le Fort I osteotomy can be used to rotate the maxilla clockwise to impact the posterior maxilla and improve incisor exposure. If the upper lip–incisor relationship is acceptable, a separate posterior segmental osteotomy can be carried out to impact the posterior maxilla and thus to achieve the desired occlusal curve. The posterior segment repositioning is determined by the posterior height of the mandibular teeth of the final occlusion. However, when the ideal posterior impaction is not aesthetically favorable or technically achievable, the mandible should be rotated counterclockwise to close the residual open bite.

CASE REPORT

Here we present a typical clinical case of a 20-year-old man with Möbius syndrome and skeletal class III malocclusion (**Fig. 7**) as a roundup of the management of VME. The patients' whole maxilla was vertically overdeveloped, especially at the posterior

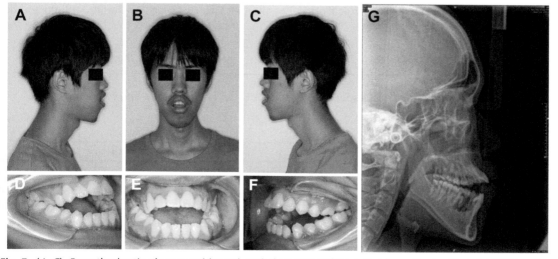

Fig. 7. (A–G). Preorthodontic photos and lateral cephalometric radiograph of a patient with total VME and an AOB of 11 mm.

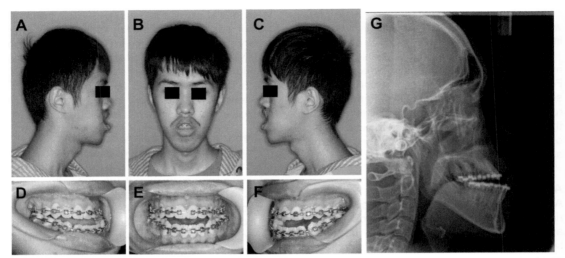

Fig. 8. (*A–G*). Presurgical photos and lateral cephalometric radiograph of a patient with an AOB of 3 mm ready for orthognathic treatment.

regions, and thus the LAFH and the mandibular plane angle was significantly increased. The maxilla was rotated counterclockwise and the mandible was rotated clockwise, and resulted in a severe anterior open bite. Owing to the long mandible, the chin was rotated to a relatively normal sagittal position. The narrow nose and palatal vaults, lip incompetence, and posterior crossbite were also observed. The gingival display was hard to evaluate because of his facial and abducens nerve palsy.

As for this patient, combination of orthodontic and orthognathic treatment was the optimal approach for correction. During the presurgical orthodontic treatment, the bilateral first premolars were extracted to create space for better alignment of the dentition. When the presurgical orthodontic treatment was completed (**Fig. 8**), clinical

examination (**Table 1**) and 2D cephalometric analysis (see **Fig. 1**) were carried out.

Based on these examinations, computer-assisted 3D surgical planning was performed (**Fig. 9**). Considering the counterclockwise rotated and vertically overdeveloped maxilla, surgical impaction and clockwise rotation were necessary. Meanwhile, the posterior crossbite of the maxillary dentition required surgical expansion for correction. A midsagittal 2-piece segmental Le Fort I osteotomy was designed to correct the vertical excess and transverse deficiency of maxilla. For a desired upper lip–incisor relationship and dentition arch, the maxilla was planned to be impacted by 6.90 mm anteriorly and 8.40 mm posteriorly of the left, as well as 7.19 mm anteriorly and 7.42 mm posteriorly of the right, whereas the

Table 1
Clinical examination findings of a patient with total VME and anterior open bite for orthognathic treatment

Items	Values
Facial ratio	Higher 66 mm; mid 63 mm; lower 76 mm
Pogonion	No deviation
Upper incisor exposure in repose	8 mm
Length of upper lip	21 mm
Nasolabial angle	Acute
Upper dental midline	1.5 mm off to right
Lower dental midline	No deviation
Canting of occlusal plane	1 mm higher on left side

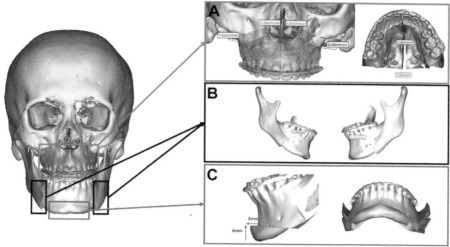

Fig. 9. Computer-assisted 3D surgical plan for midsagittal segmental Le Fort I osteotomy. (*A*) The simulation of the two-piece Le Fort I osteotomy. (*B*) The simulation of the mandibular setback procedure. (*C*) The simulation of the genioplasty and bilateral mandibular contouring.

maxilla was also planned to be expanded by 3.18 mm anteriorly and 5.19 mm posteriorly (see **Fig. 9**A). Subsequently, bilateral sagittal split ramus osteotomy (BSSRO) was planned to rotate the mandible in a counterclockwise direction and to match the terminal occlusion, where the mandible was setback by 11.52 mm on the right and 10.73 mm on the left (see **Fig. 9**B). Considering the excessive LAFH and the reduced chin prominence after mandibular setback, a genioplasty was planned for 3 mm advancement and

5 mm reduction (see **Fig. 9**C). Finally, a bilateral mandible contouring was planned for better soft tissue profile.

The orthognathic surgery and postoperative orthodontic treatment were carried out as planned, where the patient's maxilla was successfully impacted and expanded (**Fig. 10**). After postoperative orthodontic treatment, the postoperative occlusion was harmonized and maintained, with a significant improvement in the patient's profile and esthetic at the 2-year follow-up (**Fig. 11**).

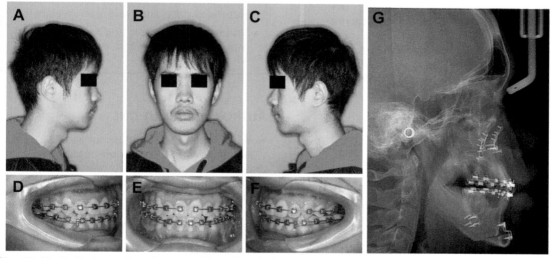

Fig. 10. (*A–G*). Postoperative photos and lateral cephalometric radiography of the same patient 3 months after orthognathic surgery.

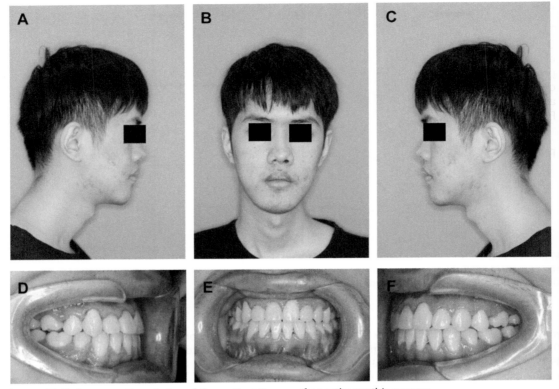

Fig. 11. (*A–F*). Postoperative photos of the patient 2 years after orthognathic surgery.

SUMMARY

Patients with different kinds of VME often show different clinical features, which requires individualized orthognathic surgical plans to correct their maxillofacial deformities. Orthognathic surgeries remain the workhorse of surgical treatment for VME and the LAFH and upper lip–incisor relationship are the key for surgical planning. The degree of bone removal and maxilla impaction depends on the extent of VME in posterior and/or anterior regions, which can be accurately simulated via computer-assisted 3D surgical planning. It is important to analyze precisely and to put forward an accurate surgical plan to normalize the deformities.

CLINICS CARE POINTS

- When managing airway after the impaction of maxilla, keep it unblocked for breath, especially nasopharyngeal cavity, and avoid acute airway obstruction.
- When reducing pain and swelling after surgery, apply cryotherapy for an average treatment time of 10–20 minutes, and avoid too rapid or prolonged cooling.
- When blood oozes from nose, carry out moderate suction and avoid swallowing blood drainage
- When eating is difficult, drink adequate fluids and avoid inadequate nutrition and dehydration.
- When intermaxillary fixation is applied for a long time, use nasogastric tube for better nutrition intake, and avoid severe weight loss.
- When nausea and vomiting occur, utilize antiemetic medications and avoid dependence on opioid analgesia.

AUTHOR CONTRIBUTIONS

H. Wu completed the manuscript text. D. He provided steps of 3D computer-assisted plan for orthognathic surgery. Y. Wu provided the orthodontic information and photos of the clinical case. L. Jiang, and X. Wang conceived the concept of this review. All authors discussed together and make comments on the study.

DECLARATION

The authors declare no competing interests.

ACKNOWLEDGMENTS

This work was supported by the National Natural Science Foundation of China (82071096), Science and Technology Commission of Shanghai Municipality (21DZ2294600), the Interdisciplinary Program of Shanghai Jiao Tong University (YG2022ZD014), and Program of Shanghai Academic/Technology Research Leader (20XD1433100).

REFERENCES

1. Naini FB, Gill DS. Orthognathic surgery. Oxford: Wiley Blackwell; 2017.
2. Angelillo JC, Dolan EA. The surgical-correction of vertical maxillary excess (long face syndrome). Ann Plas Surg 1982;8(1):64–70.
3. Reyneke JP. Essentials of orthognathic surgery. Illinois: Quintessence; 2010.
4. POSNICK JC. Orthognathic surgery: Principles & Practices. Missouri: Elsevier; 2014.
5. Tomaz A, Marinho L, Martins A, et al. Impact of orthognathic surgery on the treatment of gummy smile: an integrative review. Oral Maxillofac Surg 2020;24(3):283–8.
6. Aydil B, Ozer N, Marsan G. Facial Soft Tissue Changes after Maxillary Impaction and Mandibular Advancement in High Angle Class II Cases. Int J Med Sci 2012;9(4):316–21.
7. Fish LC, Wolford LM, Epker BN. Surgical-orthodontic correction of vertical maxillary excess. Am J Orthod Dentofac 1978;73(3):241–57.
8. Steinhaauser S, Richter U, Richter F, et al. Profile changes following maxillary impaction and autorotation of the mandible. J Orofac Orthop 2008;69(1):31–41.
9. ROSEN HM. Facial skeletal expansion - treatment strategies and rationale. Plast Reconstr Surg 1992;89(5):798–808.
10. Anehosur V, Joshi A, Nathani J, et al. Modification of LeFort I osteotomy for severe maxillary vertical excess asymmetry. Br J Oral Maxillofac Surg 2019;57(4):374–7.
11. Alkhayer A, Piffko J, Lippold C, et al. Accuracy of virtual planning in orthognathic surgery: a systematic review. Head Face Med 2020;16(1):e1–9.
12. Li BA, Wei HP, Jiang TF, et al. Randomized Clinical Trial of the Accuracy of Patient-Specific Implants versus CAD/CAM Splints in Orthognathic Surgery. Plast Reconstr Surg 2021;148(5):1101–10.
13. Chen ZX, Mo SX, Fan XM, et al. A Meta-analysis and Systematic Review Comparing the Effectiveness of Traditional and Virtual Surgical Planning for Orthognathic Surgery: Based on Randomized Clinical Trials. J Oral Maxillofac Surg 2021;79(2):e1–19.
14. Haas OL, Becker OE, de Oliveira RB. Computer-aided planning in orthognathic surgery-systematic review. Int J Oral Maxillofac Surg 2015;44(3):329–42.
15. Obwegeser H. Surgery of the maxilla for the correction of prognathism. SSO Schweiz Monatsschr Zahnheilkd 1965;75:365–74.
16. Obwegeser H. Surgical correction of small or retrodisplaced maxillae. The 'dish-face' deformity. Plast Reconstr Surg 1969;43:351–65.
17. Eshghpour M, Mianbandi V, Samieirad S. Intra- and Postoperative Complications of Le Fort I Maxillary Osteotomy. J Craniofac Surg 2018;29(8):e797–803.
18. Kramer FJ, Baethge C, Swennen G, et al. Intra- and perioperative complications of the LeFort I osteotomy: A prospective evaluation of 1000 patients. J Craniofac Surg 2004;15(6):971–7.
19. Zaroni FM, Cavalcante RC, da Costa DJ, et al. Complications associated with orthognathic surgery: A retrospective study of 485 cases. J Cranio Maxillofac Surg 2019;47(12):1855–60.
20. M W. Lehrbuch der praktischen chirurgie des mundes und der kiefer1. Leipzig: Meusser; 1935. p. 260–80.
21. Gao X, Wang T, Song JL. Orthodontic and surgical management of a patient with severe skeletal Class II deformity and facial asymmetry: A case report with a 5-year follow-up. Am J Orthod Dentofac 2017;151(4):779–92.
22. Bauer RE, Ochs MW. Maxillary Orthognathic Surgery. Oral Maxillofac Surg Clin 2014;26(4):523–31.
23. Ataoglu H, Kucukkolbasi H, Ataoglu T. Posterior segmental osteotomy of maxillary edentulous ridge: an alternative to vertical reduction. Int J Oral Maxillofac Surg 2002;31(5):558–9.
24. Philip MR. Posterior maxillary segmental osteotomy for prosthodontic rehabilitation of vertically excess maxilla -a review. J Stomatol Oral Maxi 2019;120(5):450–5.
25. Choi SK, Kwon KH. Treatment of anterior open bite by posterior maxillary segmental osteotomy and miniplates: a case report. Max Plast Reconst S 2020;42(1):e1–7.
26. Arnett GW, Bergman RT. Facial keys to orthodic dignosis and treatment planning. Am J Orthod Dentofac 1993;103(4):299–312.
27. Naini FB, Hunt NP, Moles DR. The relationship between maxillary length, differential maxillary impaction, and the change in maxillary incisor inclination. Am J Orthod Dentofac 2003;124(5):526–9.
28. Du W, Chen G, Bai D, et al. Treatment of skeletal open bite using a navigation system: CAD/CAM osteotomy and drilling guides combined with pre-bent titanium plates. Int J Oral Maxillofac Surg 2019;48(4):502–10.
29. Zahrani AA. Correction of vertical maxillary excess by superior repositioning of the maxilla. Saudi Med J 2010;31(6):695–702.

30. Hong RK, Lim SM, Heo JM, et al. Orthodontic treatment of gummy smile by maxillary total intrusion with a midpalatal absolute anchorage system. Korean J Orthod 2013;43(3):147–58.

31. Nishimura M, Sannohe M, Nagasaka H, et al. Nonextraction treatment with temporary skeletal anchorage devices to correct a Class II Division 2 malocclusion with excessive gingival display. Am J Orthod Dentofac 2014;145(1):85–94.

32. Shu R, Huang L, Bai D. Adult Class II Division 1 patient with severe gummy smile treated with temporary anchorage devices. Am J Orthod Dentofac 2011;140(1):97–105.

33. Alteneiji M, Liaw JJL, Vaid NR, et al. Treatment of VME using extra-alveolar TADs: Quantification of treatment effects. Semin Orthod 2018;24(1):123–34.

34. Hong RK, Ahn JH. Correction of a gummy smile and lip protrusion by orthodontic retreatment with lingual appliances and temporary skeletal anchorage devices. Am J Orthod Dentofac 2021;160(4):603–16.

35. Uzuka S, Chae JM, Tai K, et al. Adult gummy smile correction with temporary skeletal anchorage devices. J World Fed Orthod 2018;7(1):34–46.

Orthognathic Surgery for Obstructive Sleep Apnea

Bernadette Quah, BDS[a,b], Timothy Jie Han Sng, BDS[a,b], Chee Weng Yong, BDS, MDS(OMS)[a,b], Raymond Chung Wen Wong, BDS, MDS(OMS), PhD, FAMS[a,b,*]

KEYWORDS

- Obstructive sleep apnea • Maxillomandibular advancement • Orthognathic surgery

KEY POINTS

- Obstructive sleep apnea (OSA) is associated with comorbidities and consequences of the individual and society, and patient evaluation includes history, clinical and radiographic examination, endoscopy, and polysomnography.
- Phase II of the Stanford Protocol of surgical management involves orthognathic surgery in the form of maxillomandibular advancement (MMA).
- The surgery-first approach, adequate advancement, counterclockwise rotation, segmental surgery, or distraction osteogenesis may be beneficial in maximizing the potential of MMA.
- With good planning, MMA is effective in treating OSA, as measured with objective and subjective measures.
- Potential complications include velopharyngeal insufficiency, relapse, unsatisfactory esthetic outcomes, and poor outcomes due to the presence of medical comorbidities.

INTRODUCTION

Obstructive sleep apnea (OSA) involves obstruction (apnea) or reduction (hypopnea) of an individual's airway during sleep. OSA is defined as five or more obstructive respiratory events (apneas, hypopneas, or respiratory effort-related arousals) per hour reported on polysomnography (PSG), accompanied with symptoms such as excessive daytime sleepiness, gasping or awakening during sleep, daytime fatigue, or any associated medical disorders. An individual with ≥15 events/h with or without symptoms also fits the criteria of OSA.[1] The apnea–hypopnea index (AHI) measures the number of events of apnea or hypopnea a patient encounters per hour of sleep. The severity of OSA is classified as mild (AHI of 5 to 14), moderate (15 to 29) or severe (≥30).[2]

About 14% of men and 5% of women have an AHI ≥5, with symptoms of daytime sleepiness. This increases with increasing body mass index (BMI), age, male gender, and chronic illnesses such as cardiovascular or cerebrovascular disease and type II diabetes mellitus.[3,4]

An individual with OSA experiences fragmented sleep at night and hypersomnolence and fatigue during the day. They are more susceptible toward impairments in learning, concentration, and social interactions with depression and anxiety. Cardiovascular and cerebrovascular morbidity and mortality increases with the presence and severity of OSA. OSA is a dose-dependent risk factor for hypertension (odds ratio [OR] 2.03 to 2.89).[5] Untreated severe OSA also leads to an increase in the incidence of stroke (hazard ratio 2.86),[6] fatal and nonfatal cardiovascular events (OR 2.87 and 3.17, respectively),[7] atrial fibrillation (OR 2.18),[8] and type II diabetes mellitus (OR 2.30).[9] In addition, patients have an increased risk of

[a] Discipline of Oral and Maxillofacial Surgery, Faculty of Dentistry, National University of Singapore, Level 10, Dean's Office, National University of Oral Health Singapore, 9 Lower Kent Ridge Road, 119085, Singapore; [b] Oral and Maxillofacial Surgery, National University Centre for Oral Health Singapore
* Corresponding author. Discipline of Oral and Maxillofacial Surgery, Faculty of Dentistry, National University of Singapore, Level 10, Dean's Office, National University of Oral Health Singapore, 9 Lower Kent Ridge Road, 119085, Singapore.
E-mail address: denrwcw@nus.edu.sg

Oral Maxillofacial Surg Clin N Am 35 (2023) 49–59
https://doi.org/10.1016/j.coms.2022.06.001

perioperative complications,[2] including difficult airway intubations, respiratory depression, and longer inpatient stays.

Clinical Evaluation

Evaluation of a patient with suspected OSA begins with a detailed sleep history, for example, snoring, gasping, choking, witnessed apneas, excessive sleepiness, total amount of sleep, nocturia, headaches, sleep fragmentation, and decreased concentration or memory.[10] An evaluation of potential or reported comorbidities and risk factors should also be documented.

The Epworth Sleepiness Scale (ESS), Berlin Questionnaire, STOP-BANG scoring, and OSA-50 questionnaire are questionnaires that aid in determining a patient's OSA risk, but should not be used alone to diagnose OSA.[4]

Patients are evaluated for obesity using BMI, large neck circumference (>16 to 17 inches), craniofacial (eg, retrognathia), and nasal abnormalities (eg, turbinate hypertrophy, septal deviation). The oral cavity is examined for increased incisal overjet, a narrow high-arched palate, and macroglossia. Patients with upper airway narrowing may present with an enlarged uvula or soft palate, narrow lateral pharyngeal wall, or tonsillar hypertrophy. The Mallampati and Friedman tongue position scores may aid evaluation of a crowded airway.[10]

Imaging is useful in the evaluation of a patient's airway. Lateral cephalometry evaluates skeletal discrepancies, posterior airway space (PAS), soft palate length, or an inferiorly positioned hyoid.[11] Computed tomography allows good soft tissue contrast, precise measurements of cross-sectional airway areas, and three-dimensional reconstruction, whereas magnetic resonance imaging provides dynamic airway evaluation and detailed evaluation of various types of soft tissues without radiation exposure.[12]

Nasoendoscopy allows direct visualization of the mechanism of snoring and the site of airway obstruction. Drug-induced sleep endoscopy (DISE) is shown to predict if a patient responds positively to upper airway surgery—nonresponders showed a higher frequency of circumferential collapse at the velum and antero-posterior collapse at the tongue base or epiglottis.[13]

The home sleep apnea test has recently been introduced as a simpler alternative to diagnose OSA in "less complicated" individuals. Sleep study with PSG, however, remains the gold standard for diagnosis of OSA.[4]

Treatment

Nonsurgical management for OSA includes weight loss, continuous positive airway pressure (CPAP) therapy, and mandibular advancement devices. However, these strategies have limitations.[14] Weight loss is challenging for patients with OSA, whereas CPAP requires good patient compliance as patients may not tolerate the side effects (eg, mask discomfort, rhinorrhea, dry mouth, nasal congestion, aerophagia, and conjunctivitis) and more than 50% eventually refuse CPAP.[15] Mandibular advancement devices too have adverse effects such as sialorrhea, temporomandibular joint pain, tooth discomfort, and malocclusion.

Surgical management of OSA aims to correct or reduce anatomic factors that contribute to airway obstruction. The Stanford Protocol is a guideline for the surgical assessment and management of the patient with OSA (**Fig. 1**).[16]

The extent of surgery depends on the severity and location of airway obstruction. Nasal surgeries aid in eliminating nasal passage obstructions that result in patients breathing through their mouth when sleeping and their tongue subsequently falling posteriorly to obstruct the airway. Tongue or palate surgeries reduce airway obstruction caused by anatomic variations in their respective sites of the pharynx.

Maxillomandibular Advancement

Maxillomandibular advancement (MMA) incorporates the surgical techniques used for orthognathic surgery. Maxillary advancement with a Le Fort I osteotomy moves the hard and soft palates and velopharyngeal muscles anteriorly to open the airway. With a ramus osteotomy, mandibular advancement especially combined with genioplasty advancement, pulls forward the tongue and suprahyoid muscles. Adjunctive procedures (eg, septoplasty, hard palate advancement) can be done concurrently to remove other potential sources of airway obstruction.

In the original Stanford Protocol, MMA was considered Phase II surgery; only patients in whom OSA failed to improve after Phase I surgery would be considered for MMA. The investigators have proven the immense success of MMA without Phase I surgery first.[17] In response, the 2019 guideline expanded the indications for Phase II surgery without Phase I to include:

1. Patients with OSA having dentofacial deformities or other indications for orthognathic surgery
2. Moderate to severe patients with OSA having anatomic findings that Phase I surgery would not result in significant improvement:
   a. Complete lateral pharyngeal wall collapse on DISE

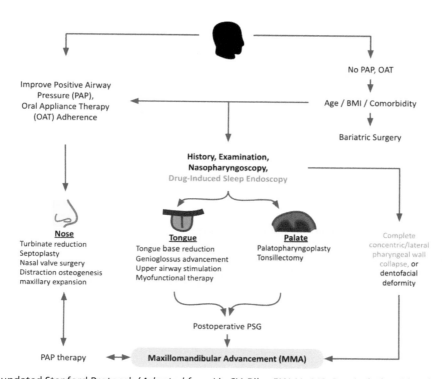

Fig. 1. The updated Stanford Protocol. (*Adapted from* Liu SY, Riley RW, Yu MS. Surgical Algorithm for Obstructive Sleep Apnea: An Update. *Clin Exp Otorhinolaryngol.* 2020;13(3):215-224.)

    b. Low hyoid position and obtuse cervicomental angle

    c. High occlusal plane inclination

SURGICAL CONSIDERATIONS

The surgical considerations for orthognathic surgery for skeletal discrepancies are well-documented and are applicable for the management of OSA. However, accompanying comorbidities and airway-related considerations warrant specific considerations for MMA, which are discussed below.

Timing of Surgery

Patients with OSA may benefit from a surgery-first or surgery-early approach (SFA). The conventional approach of orthodontic decompensation before MMA may provide a more optimal postsurgical occlusion. However, this increases the duration for resolution of OSA symptoms and may even transiently aggravate them.[18] Patients may thus still require CPAP therapy while undergoing presurgical orthodontics.

    SFA, on the other hand, promptly attenuates apnea-related symptoms and comorbid diseases by expanding the airway and correcting any skeletal discrepancies. The regional acceleratory phenomenon allows more efficient postsurgical orthodontic movement that reduces overall treatment time.[19] Hence, patient satisfaction rates are high.[20] An SFA may even be indicated if the postoperative occlusion is reasonable and stable, and if the patient does not want or cannot afford orthodontics.

    Potential concerns regarding SFA include the need for greater surgical movements, as well as postsurgical instability, although its influence on relapse is not well studied. Nonetheless, with good patient selection, judicious collaboration, and precise planning, predictable good outcomes from SFA may soon be the norm.

Degree of Movement

Strong evidence is lacking regarding a minimum amount of maxillary or mandibular advancement for optimal treatment outcomes. A mandibular advancement of 10 mm is commonly advocated.[21-23] However, a systematic review and meta-analysis by Holty and Guilleminault found that a greater degree of maxillary (9.5 mm) instead of mandibular advancement was associated with surgical success in patients with OSA.[24]

Counterclockwise Rotation

Counterclockwise rotation (CCWR) of the maxillo-mandibular complex provides both functional and esthetic advantages for management of OSA.[25,26] CCWR maximizes the advancement of the base of tongue and suprahyoid muscles and brings the soft palate downward and forward. Mehra and colleagues reported a significant increase in the PAS in lateral cephalometric radiographs at these regions when CCWR was performed.[27] CCWR also normalizes the facial profile of patients with high mandibular plane angles[25] and can be a stable procedure when executed judiciously.[28,29]

Future prospective clinical trials are still required to ascertain the degree of rotation required, and whether it results in greater surgical cure or success when compared with MMA alone in patients with OSA.[30]

Segmental Surgery

Modifications to the conventional Le Fort I and ramus osteotomies via segmental surgeries are useful in some instances[26,31]:

1. Coordination of the dental arches
2. Expansion of a narrow maxillary arch with a maxillary midline split
3. Esthetic considerations

Large advancements may result an elevated nasal tip or fullness of the cheeks and paranasal regions, leading to an unesthetic bimaxillary protrusive or "simian" appearance.[32] This is especially of concern in patients with a normal sagittal profile or preexisting bimaxillary protrusion, such as in oriental populations. In these patients, anterior segmental osteotomies may be considered for retraction of the anterior segments to prevent this profile change (Fig. 2). In situations where previous extractions have been performed, we need to balance maximal advancement and facial appearance, making use of methods such as CCWR and maxillary impaction (Fig. 3).

However, one must take into consideration the potential complications of segmental surgery. Patients with OSA having medical comorbidities may not be able to tolerate the increased physiologic burden caused by the increased duration of surgery. Segmental surgery also increases the potential risk for damage to the adjacent teeth as well as ischemia of a multi-segmented jaw.

Genioplasty Advancement

Genioplasty advancement moves the genial tubercle, genioglossus, and geniohyoid muscles forward to enlarge the retroglossal space and may be considered in patients with base of tongue obstructions. Genioplasty alone was reported to result in a 67.8% of reduction in AHI.[15] In combination with MMA, this gives greater advancement of the genial tubercle. This is also beneficial esthetically in patients with a retruded or small chin.

Distraction osteogenesis

In addition to conventional orthognathic surgery, distraction osteogenesis may also be considered for the management of OSA especially if larger advancements are needed (Fig. 4). Tables 1 and 2 provide a comparison between conventional orthognathic surgery versus mandibular distraction osteogenesis and maxillary transverse expansion with distraction osteogenesis, respectively.[33–37]

EFFECTIVENESS OF MAXILLOMANDIBULAR ADVANCEMENT

The outcome of each intervention for OSA is evaluated by the success and complication rate. PSG is also used to measure the success of the prescribed OSA treatment, apart from diagnosis.[38] Common PSG parameters include the AHI, respiratory disturbance index (RDI), and lowest oxygen saturation (Lsat). Treatment success is defined as an AHI or RDI less than 20 with at least 50% of reduction from the initial index, whereas cure is defined as an AHI or RDI less than 5.[23,39,40]

There is undeniable evidence that MMA is effective in improving the AHI, RDI, and Lsat levels in patients with OSA. Meta-analyses have reported mean reductions of AHI and RDI by 44.76 to 47.8 and 44.4 to 59.7, respectively. Similarly, Lsat levels improved by a mean of 10.8 to 16.9.[24,41,42] With reported success and cure rates of 85.5% to 100% and 38.5% to 43.2%, respectively, MMA proves to be an important tool in the treatment of OSA with long-term stability.[43]

Although PSG remains the standard modality of objectively assessing treatment outcomes, it may not be sufficient in evaluating subjective changes. Questionnaires or quality of life (QOL) instruments assess patient-reported outcomes of MMA[44] and include the ESS, excessive daytime somnolence (EDS) or simply on how snoring has affected the patient's bed partner.[45] MMA resulted in marked improvement or complete resolution of an EDS scores in patients with profound EDS and moderate to severe snoring habits. Furthermore, 80% of the patients no longer snored, whereas the remaining 20% became mild snorers.[23] Significant improvements in ESS scores after MMA were demonstrated by multiple investigators.[24,41,42]

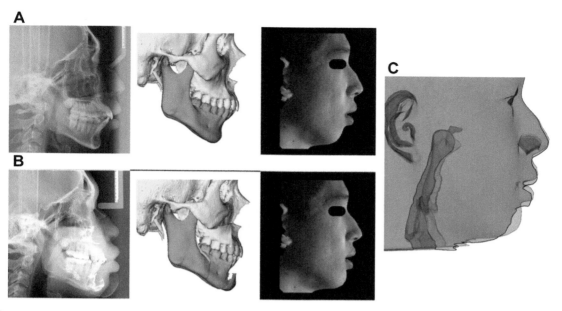

Fig. 2. Preoperative (*A*) and postoperative (*B*) lateral cephalogram, bony and soft tissue simulation of an OSA patient with bimaxillary protrusion (*A*). Maxillary and mandibular anterior segmental osteotomies were planned to prevent exacerbation of his bimaxillary protrusion. Three-dimensional planning also allows simulation of changes to the airway (*C*).

Lye and colleagues reported a 93.3% improvement in QOL postoperatively, with an average postoperative Functional Outcomes of Sleep Questionnaire (FOSQ) score of ≥18, indicating normal functional status.[46] However, there was no correlation between the FOSQ and PSG parameters. In contrast, Butterfield and colleagues reported that the changes in AHI correlated significantly with the Obstructive Sleep Apnea Questionnaire (OSA-18). These differences may result from the varying dimensions evaluated by the various QOL instruments.

Authors have also attempted to correlate radiographic changes with improvement in OSA. Riley and colleagues measured the PAS via lateral cephalometry preoperatively and postoperatively and reported an enlargement of 6.4 ± 0.5 mm after surgery but failed to establish a relationship between PAS and PSG.[23] The effectiveness of two-dimensional cephalometry in evaluating treatment outcomes therefore may not adequately replicate the three-dimensional changes in the airway.[47]

Consequentially, some have employed the use of cone-beam computed tomography to provide a three-dimensional representation of the upper airway.[48–50] Veys and colleagues reported an increase in the total airway volume by 35.4% after MMA (from 28,780 to 38,970 mm³). The oropharyngeal airway volume in particular attained a significant increase of 80.2% (from 7641 to 13,770 mm³); this increase correlated with improvements in the patients' AHI.

Apart from surrogate measurements of the airway, some have explored direct assessment of physical changes in the airway via endoscopy. Using DISE, Liu and colleagues evaluated patients' dynamic airway changes before and after MMA and noted the most significant improvements in airway collapse at the lateral pharyngeal wall.[51] The patients with the most improvement in lateral pharyngeal wall collapsibility also demonstrated the largest changes in the AHI (from 60.0 to 7.5).

COMPLICATIONS OF MAXILLOMANDIBULAR ADVANCEMENT

MMA possesses the same potential complications as orthognathic surgery for other indications.[52–54] This includes planning errors, hemorrhage, neurosensory disturbances, unfavorable fractures, oroantral communication, dental injury, infection, ischemia of osteotomy segments, malocclusion, temporomandibular joint dysfunction, fixation failure, or malunion.

With large surgical movements and a frequent need for adjunctive surgical procedures, MMA for OSA may theoretically be at greater risk for complications as compared with the typical orthognathic surgery. Fortunately, complication

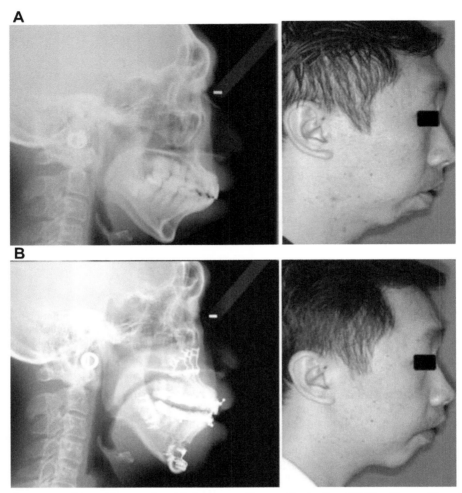

Fig. 3. Previous upper bicuspid extraction (*A*) for camouflage orthodontics. CCWR with maxillary impaction, MMA and genioplasty (*B*) done, balancing medical necessity of MMA with facial appearance. Pogonion advanced 24 mm.

rates are low across studies, with a minor and major complication rate of 3.1% and 1.0%, respectively.[24,41,42] A mean period of 3.5 days of hospitalization has been reported across the studies. MMA is considered a safe surgical procedure, with no reported deaths, although Zaghi and colleagues suggest that any deaths may simply be unpublished.[41]

Four specific concerns for MMA in patients with OSA are discussed below:

1. Velopharyngeal Insufficiency

   Velopharyngeal insufficiency (VPI) has been reported after Le Fort I advancement,[23] particularly in patients with a history of cleft palate.[55,56] This predisposition to VPI may be due to an already compromised soft palate architecture, or the large maxillary advancements often required in cleft patients.[55–57] Similarly, patients with OSA who planned for MMA may have had or need soft palate surgery (ie, uvulopalatopharyngoplasty) and also require significant maxillary advancement. The incidence of VPI after MMA ranges substantially by study from 0% to 100%.[24,47,58–60] As expected, VPI was mostly reported in MMA patients who also had palatal surgeries.[23,56] Fortunately, a majority of the VPI could be resolved with speech therapy, without any further surgical intervention.[58,60]

2. Relapse

   The postoperative stability of MMA is thought to be potentially hindered by traction or pressure from the stretched surrounding

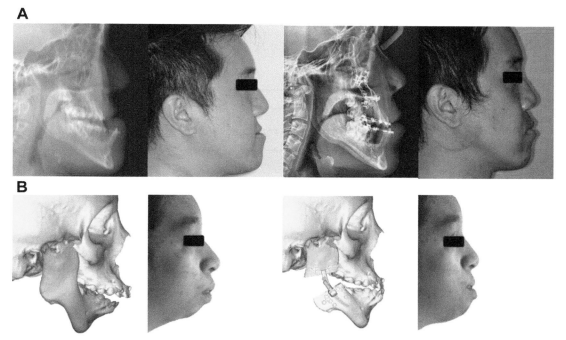

Fig. 4. Distraction osteogenesis done for maxilla (*A*: advanced 18 mm) and mandible (*B*: advanced 20 mm) for better stability.

soft tissues, poor bone contact between segments, and inadequate rigidity of fixation.[61] Using a 0.5 mm or 1° deviation to determine surgical relapse, multiple investigators have concluded that despite the large surgical movements required for MMA, stability was still well achieved.[23,62–64] This was attributed to the use of rigid internal fixation and skeletal suspension techniques.[65,66]

3. Unsatisfactory Esthetic Outcome

As discussed earlier, large surgical movements may significantly change the patient's facial profile leading to dissatisfaction with their postoperative appearance.

Table 1
Distraction osteogenesis versus sagittal split osteotomy for mandibular advancement in patients with obstructive sleep apnea

Mandibular Distraction Osteogenesis	Bilateral Sagittal Split Osteotomy
Average distraction distance: 12–29 mm	Advocated advancement: 10 mm

Adults
  Success rate: 100%
  Cure rates: 82%–100%
  Infant: not defined, no clear reported rates
	Adults
	  Success rate: 86%
	  Cure rate: 43.2%

Relapse
  Not significantly different from bilateral sagittal split osteotomy (BSSO)
	Relapse
	  10%–20% relapse in up to 15% after MMA, but without associated symptoms or worsening of the AHI

Age
  Apt option to lengthen the mandible in children (especially in syndromic cases) to open the airway
	Age
	  Usually not performed in pediatric patients due to the presence of developing tooth buds and continual growth of the facial skeleton

Data from Refs.[33,34]

Table 2
Distraction osteogenesis versus segmental Le Fort I surgery for maxillary transverse expansion in patients with obstructive sleep apnea

Distraction Osteogenesis	Segmental Le Fort I Osteotomy
Up to 12 mm of expansion	Typically, 5–7 mm of expansion
Stability Less stability for segmental Le Fort I osteotomy as compared with maxillary transverse distraction osteogenesis	
Relapse 4%–8% at intercanine distance 3%–8% at intermolar distance	Relapse 5%–25% at intercanine distance 20%–50% at intermolar distance
Need for second surgery (segmental osteotomy) to correct any antero-posterior (AP), vertical discrepancy, yaw, pitch, and cant	Greater control and arrangement of segments in all 3 dimensions and 6 planes of space in the same surgical setting
Ability to create space/relieve crowding of the arch	
Creation of midline diastema in the initial phase that may be unesthetic	May not involve creation of midline diastema

Data from Refs.[35–37]

A strong correlation between dentofacial deformities, especially mandibular retrognathia and OSA has been reported.[67] A study of patient-reported outcomes found that 86% of patients felt their appearance improved after surgery for mandibular retrognathia.[68] However, 8.21% of patients were disappointed with their appearance after MMA[42]; this dissatisfaction was higher in younger patients and those with a thinner soft tissue profile.[69]

It is therefore imperative for patient counseling on potential facial changes. These changes can be simulated virtually, keeping in mind the limitations and inaccuracies of the simulation[70] (see **Fig. 2**).

4. Medical Comorbidities

Patients with OSA typically seek treatment at an older age and often present with comorbidities such as hypertension, diabetes mellitus, or a high BMI. As a result, the patient may be at higher risk of major complications such as cardiac arrest, dysrhythmia, or poor wound healing. Therefore, surgeons must be mindful to optimize the patient's medical conditions preoperatively.[24,41,42]

SUMMARY

The indications and considerations of orthognathic surgery for the management of OSA are constantly evolving. Despite the greater surgical movements and associated comorbidities in patients with OSA, MMA has been proven to be a safe and effective modality of treatment, although we should all strive to reduce complications with better planning, execution, and communication.

CLINICS CARE POINTS

- Revised guidelines indicate the advantages of early Phase II maxillomandibular advancement (MMA) and other surgical adjuncts in patients with obstructive sleep apnea (OSA) with concomitant dentofacial deformities. There are no clear advantages in trying other Phase I methods first in these cases.

- The medical necessity of adequate MMA will need to be balanced with the effects on facial appearance. Selectively using counterclockwise rotation with maxillary impaction and MMA, combined with advancement genioplasty (incorporating the genial tubercle) may be needed to maximize the advancement.

- A presurgical protrusive facial appearance might necessitate consideration of segmental surgery if the soft tissues are unable to accommodate single piece advancement.
- Presurgical orthodontics might be needed for adequate decompensation and maximize surgical movement. In moderate to severe OSA cases, such patients undergoing presurgical orthodontics will need to be on continuous positive airway pressure therapy to avoid adverse events while waiting for surgery.

DISCLOSURE

The authors have nothing to disclose.

CONFLICT OF INTEREST

None of the authors have any conflict of interest, financial or otherwise. No funding was received.

REFERENCES

1. Sateia MJ. International classification of sleep disorders-third edition: highlights and modifications. Chest 2014;146(5):1387–94.
2. Park JG, Ramar K, Olson EJ. Updates on definition, consequences, and management of obstructive sleep apnea. Mayo Clin Proc 2011;86(6):549–55.
3. Peppard PE, Young T, Barnet JH, et al. Increased prevalence of sleep-disordered breathing in adults. Am J Epidemiol 2013;177(9):1006–14.
4. Kapur VK, Auckley DH, Chowdhuri S, et al. Clinical Practice Guideline for Diagnostic Testing for Adult Obstructive Sleep Apnea: An American Academy of Sleep Medicine Clinical Practice Guideline. J Clin Sleep Med 2017;13(3):479–504.
5. Peppard PE, Young T, Palta M, et al. Prospective study of the association between sleep-disordered breathing and hypertension. N Engl J Med 2000; 342(19):1378–84.
6. Redline S, Yenokyan G, Gottlieb DJ, et al. Obstructive sleep apnea-hypopnea and incident stroke: the sleep heart health study. Am J Respir Crit Care Med 2010;182(2):269–77.
7. Marin JM, Carrizo SJ, Vicente E, et al. Long-term cardiovascular outcomes in men with obstructive sleep apnea-hypopnea with or without treatment with continuous positive airway pressure: an observational study. Lancet 2005;365(9464):1046–53.
8. Gami AS, Hodge DO, Herges RM, et al. Obstructive sleep apnea, obesity, and the risk of incident atrial fibrillation. J Am Coll Cardiol 2007;49(5):565–71.

9. Reichmuth KJ, Austin D, Skatrud JB, et al. Association of sleep apnea and type II diabetes: a population-based study. Am J Respir Crit Care Med 2005;172(12):1590–5.
10. Epstein LJ, Kristo D, Strollo PJ Jr, et al. Clinical guideline for the evaluation, management and long-term care of obstructive sleep apnea in adults. J Clin Sleep Med 2009;5(3):263–76.
11. Riley R, Guilleminault C, Herran J, et al. Cephalometric analyses and flow-volume loops in obstructive sleep apnea patients. Sleep 1983;6(4):303–11.
12. Stuck BA, Maurer JT. Airway evaluation in obstructive sleep apnea. Sleep Med Rev 2008;12(6): 411–36.
13. Koutsourelakis I, Safiruddin F, Ravesloot M, et al. Surgery for obstructive sleep apnea: sleep endoscopy determinants of outcome. Laryngoscope 2012;122(11):2587–91.
14. Faber J, Faber C, Faber AP. Obstructive sleep apnea in adults. Dental Press J Orthod 2019;24(3): 99–109.
15. Holty JE, Guilleminault C. Surgical options for the treatment of obstructive sleep apnea. Med Clin North Am 2010;94(3):479–515.
16. Liu SY, Awad M, Riley R, et al. The Role of the Revised Stanford Protocol in Today's Precision Medicine. Sleep Med Clin 2019;14(1):99–107.
17. Boyd SB, Walters AS, Song Y, et al. Comparative effectiveness of maxillomandibular advancement and uvulopalatopharyngoplasty for the treatment of moderate to severe obstructive sleep apnea. J Oral Maxillofac Surg 2013;71(4):743–51.
18. Kim S-J, Kim KB. Orthodontics in obstructive sleep apnea patients. Chapter 7. Springer Nature Swizterland AG; 2020. p. 81–95.
19. Jung J, Moon SH, Kwon YD. Current status of surgery-first approach (part III): the use of 3D technology and the implication in obstructive sleep apnea. Maxillofac Plast Reconstr Surg 2020;42(1):1.
20. Peiró-Guijarro MA, Guijarro-Martínez R, Hernández-Alfaro F. Surgery first in orthognathic surgery: A systematic review of the literature. Am J Orthod Dentofacial Orthop 2016;149(4):448–62.
21. Hochban W, Brandenburg U, Peter JH. Surgical treatment of obstructive sleep apnea by maxillomandibular advancement. Sleep 1994;17(7):624–9.
22. Reiche-Fischel O, Wolford LM. Posterior airway space changes after double jaw surgery with counter-clockwise rotation. AAOMS 78th Annual Meeting and Scientific Sessions. J Oral Maxillofac Surg 1996;54:96.
23. Riley RW, Powell NB, Li KK, et al. Surgery and obstructive sleep apnea: long-term clinical outcomes. Otolaryngol Head Neck Surg 2000;122(3): 415–21.
24. Holty JE, Guilleminault C. Maxillomandibular advancement for the treatment of obstructive sleep

apnea: a systematic review and meta-analysis. Sleep Med Rev 2010;14(5):287–97.

25. Lee WJ, Hwang DH, Liu SY, et al. Subtypes of Maxillomandibular Advancement Surgery for Patients With Obstructive Sleep Apnea. J Craniofac Surg 2016;27(8):1965–70.

26. Cheng-Hui Lin C, Wang PF, Ray Han Loh S, et al. Maxillomandibular Rotational Advancement: Airway, Aesthetics, and Angle's Considerations. Sleep Med Clin 2019;14(1):83–9.

27. Mehra P, Downie M, Pita MC, et al. Pharyngeal airway space changes after counterclockwise rotation of the maxillomandibular complex. Am J Orthod Dentofacial Orthop 2001;120(2):154–9.

28. Wolford LM, Chemello PD, Hilliard F. Occlusal plane alteration in orthognathic surgery–Part I: Effects on function and esthetics. Am J Orthod Dentofacial Orthop 1994;106(3):304–16.

29. Chemello PD, Wolford LM, Buschang PH. Occlusal plane alteration in orthognathic surgery–Part II: Long-term stability of results. Am J Orthod Dentofacial Orthop 1994;106(4):434–40.

30. Knudsen TB, Laulund AS, Ingerslev J, et al. Improved apnea-hypopnea index and lowest oxygen saturation after maxillomandibular advancement with or without counterclockwise rotation in patients with obstructive sleep apnea: a meta-analysis. J Oral Maxillofac Surg 2015;73(4):719–26.

31. Liao YF, Chiu YT, Lin CH, et al. Modified maxillomandibular advancement for obstructive sleep apnea: towards a better outcome for Asians. Int J Oral Maxillofac Surg 2015;44(2):189–94.

32. Powers DB, Allan PF, Hayes CJ, et al. A review of the surgical treatment options for the obstructive sleep apnea/hypopnea syndrome patient. Mil Med 2010; 175(9):676–85.

33. Tsui WK, Yang Y, Cheung LK, et al. Distraction osteogenesis as a treatment of obstructive sleep apnea syndrome: A systematic review. Medicine (Baltimore) 2016;95(36):e4674.

34. Tsui WK, Yang Y, Mcgrath C, et al. Mandibular distraction osteogenesis versus sagittal split ramus osteotomy in managing obstructive sleep apnea: A randomized clinical trial. J Craniomaxillofac Surg 2019;47(5):750–7.

35. Conley RS, Legan HL. Correction of severe obstructive sleep apnea with bimaxillary transverse distraction osteogenesis and maxillomandibular advancement. Am J Orthod Dentofacial Orthop 2006;129(2):283–92.

36. Silverstein K, Quinn PD. Surgically-assisted rapid palatal expansion for management of transverse maxillary deficiency. J Oral Maxillofac Surg 1997; 55(7):725–7.

37. Bailey LJ, White RP Jr, Proffit WR, et al. Segmental Le Fort I osteotomy for management of transverse maxillary deficiency. J Oral Maxillofac Surg 1997; 55(7):728–31.

38. Douglas NJ, Thomas S, Jan MA. Clinical value of polysomnography. Lancet 1992;339(8789):347–50.

39. Sher AE. Upper airway surgery for obstructive sleep apnea. Sleep Med Rev 2002;6(3):195–212.

40. Thakkar K, Yao M. Diagnostic studies in obstructive sleep apnea. Otolaryngol Clin North Am 2007;40(4): 785–805.

41. Zaghi S, Holty JE, Certal V, et al. Maxillomandibular Advancement for Treatment of Obstructive Sleep Apnea: A Meta-analysis. JAMA Otolaryngol Head Neck Surg 2016;142(1):58–66.

42. John CR, Gandhi S, Sakharia AR, et al. Maxillomandibular advancement is a successful treatment for obstructive sleep apnea: a systematic review and meta-analysis. Int J Oral Maxillofac Surg 2018; 47(12):1561–71.

43. Camacho M, Noller MW, Del Do M, et al. Long-term Results for Maxillomandibular Advancement to Treat Obstructive Sleep Apnea: A Meta-analysis. Otolaryngol Head Neck Surg 2019;160(4):580–93.

44. Parish JM, Lyng PJ. Quality of life in bed partners of patients with obstructive sleep apnea or hypopnea after treatment with continuous positive airway pressure. Chest 2003;124(3):942–7.

45. Goodday RH, Bourque SE, Edwards PB. Objective and Subjective Outcomes Following Maxillomandibular Advancement Surgery for Treatment of Patients With Extremely Severe Obstructive Sleep Apnea (Apnea-Hypopnea Index >100). J Oral Maxillofac Surg 2016;74(3):583–9.

46. Lye KW, Waite PD, Meara D, et al. Quality of life evaluation of maxillomandibular advancement surgery for treatment of obstructive sleep apnea. J Oral Maxillofac Surg 2008;66(5):968–72.

47. Smatt Y, Ferri J. Retrospective study of 18 patients treated by maxillomandibular advancement with adjunctive procedures for obstructive sleep apnea syndrome. J Craniofac Surg 2005;16(5):770–7.

48. Veys B, Pottel L, Mollemans W, et al. Three-dimensional volumetric changes in the upper airway after maxillomandibular advancement in obstructive sleep apnea patients and the impact on quality of life. Int J Oral Maxillofac Surg 2017;46(12):1525–32.

49. Bianchi A, Betti E, Tarsitano A, et al. Volumetric three-dimensional computed tomographic evaluation of the upper airway in patients with obstructive sleep apnea syndrome treated by maxillomandibular advancement. Br J Oral Maxillofac Surg 2014; 52(9):831–7.

50. Fairburn SC, Waite PD, Vilos G, et al. Three-dimensional changes in upper airways of patients with obstructive sleep apnea following maxillomandibular advancement. J Oral Maxillofac Surg 2007; 65(1):6–12.

51. Liu SY, Huon LK, Powell NB, et al. Lateral Pharyngeal Wall Tension After Maxillomandibular Advancement for Obstructive Sleep Apnea Is a Marker for Surgical Success: Observations From Drug-Induced Sleep Endoscopy. J Oral Maxillofac Surg 2015;73(8):1575–82.

52. Robl MT, Farrell BB, Tucker MR. Complications in orthognathic surgery: a report of 1,000 cases. Oral Maxillofac Surg Clin North Am 2014;26(4):599–609.

53. Kim YK. Complications associated with orthognathic surgery. J Korean Assoc Oral Maxillofac Surg 2017; 43(1):3–15.

54. Sousa CS, Turrini RN. Complications in orthognathic surgery: A comprehensive review. J Oral Maxillofac Surg Med Pathol 2012;24:67–74.

55. McComb RW, Marrinan EM, Nuss RC, et al. Predictors of velopharyngeal insufficiency after Le Fort I maxillary advancement in patients with cleft palate. J Oral Maxillofac Surg 2011;69(8):2226–32.

56. Wu Y, Wang X, Ma L, et al. Velopharyngeal Configuration Changes Following Le Fort I Osteotomy With Maxillary Advancement in Patients With Cleft Lip and Palate: A Cephalometric Study. Cleft Palate Craniofac J 2015;52(6):711–6.

57. Chanchareonsook N, Samman N, Whitehill TL. The effect of cranio-maxillofacial osteotomies and distraction osteogenesis on speech and velopharyngeal status: a critical review. Cleft Palate Craniofac J 2006;43(4):477–87.

58. Li KK, Troell RJ, Riley RW, et al. Uvulopalatopharyngoplasty, maxillomandibular advancement, and the velopharynx. Laryngoscope 2001;111(6):1075–8.

59. Hendler BH, Costello BJ, Silverstein K, et al. A protocol for uvulopalatopharyngoplasty, mortised genioplasty, and maxillomandibular advancement in patients with obstructive sleep apnea: an analysis of 40 cases. J Oral Maxillofac Surg 2001;59(8):892–9.

60. Bettega G, Pépin JL, Veale D, et al. Obstructive sleep apnea syndrome. fifty-one consecutive patients treated by maxillofacial surgery. Am J Respir Crit Care Med 2000;162(2 Pt 1):641–9.

61. Proffit WR, Turvey TA, Phillips C. The hierarchy of stability and predictability in orthognathic surgery with rigid fixation: an update and extension. Head Face Med 2007;3:21.

62. Li KK, Powell NB, Riley RW, et al. Long-Term Results of Maxillomandibular Advancement Surgery. Sleep Breath 2000;4(3):137–40.

63. Bothur S, Blomqvist JE, Isaksson S. Stability of Le Fort I osteotomy with advancement: a comparison of single maxillary surgery and a two-jaw procedure. J Oral Maxillofac Surg 1998;56(9):1029–34.

64. Lee SH, Kaban LB, Lahey ET. Skeletal stability of patients undergoing maxillomandibular advancement for treatment of obstructive sleep apnea. J Oral Maxillofac Surg 2015;73(4):694–700.

65. Ellis E 3rd, Gallo WJ. Relapse following mandibular advancement with dental plus skeletal maxillomandibular fixation. J Oral Maxillofac Surg 1986;44(7):509–15.

66. Van Sickels JE. A comparative study of bicortical screws and suspension wires versus bicortical screws in large mandibular advancements. J Oral Maxillofac Surg 1991;49(12):1293–8.

67. Posnick JC, Adachie A, Singh N, et al. Silent" Sleep Apnea in Dentofacial Deformities and Prevalence of Daytime Sleepiness After Orthognathic and Intranasal Surgery. J Oral Maxillofac Surg 2018;76(4):833–43.

68. Aubry C, Bouchard C, Paris M, et al. Satisfaction with Facial Appearance following Bimaxillary Orthognathic Surgery. J Oral Maxillofac Surg 2021;79(10 Suppl):e19–20.

69. Li KK, Riley RW, Powell NB, et al. Patient's perception of the facial appearance after maxillomandibular advancement for obstructive sleep apnea syndrome. J Oral Maxillofac Surg 2001;59(4):377–81.

70. Lee KJC, Tan SL, Low HYA, et al. Accuracy of 3-dimensional soft tissue prediction for orthognathic surgery in a Chinese population. J Stomatol Oral Maxillofac Surg 2021. https://doi.org/10.1016/j.jormas.2021.08.001. S2468-7855(21)00161-0.

Patient-Specific Implants in Orthognathic Surgery

Dion Tik Shun Li, BSc, DMD, MDS[a], Yiu Yan Leung, BDS, MDS, PhD[a],*

KEYWORDS

- Orthognathic surgery • Dentofacial deformity • Virtual surgical planning • 3D printing
- Patient-specific implant • Accuracy

KEY POINTS

- Conventional orthognathic surgery using a wafer-based approach has limitations and potential errors in various steps of the procedure.
- Virtual surgical planning and three-dimensional printing allow the concept of a waferless approach by patient-specific implant (PSI).
- PSI has proved to be accurate in the execution of the planned movement of the orthognathic procedures.
- There are pros and cons of using PSI as a routine in orthognathic surgery.
- Further development and improvement of PSI as well as an increase in popularity of its use in the near future are expected.

INTRODUCTION

When asked what is *the* breakthrough of the decade in orthognathic surgery, perhaps most surgeons would agree that it is the development of virtual surgical planning (VSP) combined with personalized cutting guides and fixation plates, known in the field as patient-specific implants (PSI). Although the importance of chairside clinical assessment remains unchanged in the presurgical workup, the use of three-dimensional (3D) imaging, surgical simulation software, and 3D printing technology has been rapidly implemented in the past decade to enhance certainty in surgical planning, precision in operative execution, and predictability of the outcome. The popularity of PSI in orthognathic surgery has continued to increase in recent years, because of its reported accuracy and ability to overcome many of the limitations of the conventional approaches, such as reliance on the rotational path of the temporomandibular joint (TMJ) and opposing occlusion. In this article, we discuss the development from conventional orthognathic surgery to VSP, translating the virtual plan to the patient from a wafer-based- to a waferless approach using PSI, technical aspects of PSI design and fabrication, accuracy and pros and cons of PSI, and future directions in the field.

CONVENTIONAL ORTHOGNATHIC APPROACH

During conventional orthognathic planning, decisions on the movements of surgical jaw repositioning are made based on 2D radiographic examination, as well as dental model analysis, after clinical assessment. Soft tissue changes in 2D after the planned bony repositioning are predicted either by manual cephalometric tracing or by computer programs that merge tracings of cephalograms to preoperative photographs of the patients. After this initial preparation stage, the next step would be to utilize a system that reliably translates surgical planning to the actual surgery.

The development of the method for translating surgical planning to the patient was adopted from our dental background, as the conventional approach relies on the facebow/articulator system. Stone dental casts are mounted in a 3D position replicating their position in relation to the rest

[a] Oral and Maxillofacial Surgery, Faculty of Dentistry, The University of Hong Kong, Hong Kong
* Corresponding author. Oral and Maxillofacial Surgery, Prince Philip Dental Hospital, 34 Hospital Road, Hong Kong.
E-mail address: mikeyyleung@hku.hk

Oral Maxillofacial Surg Clin N Am 35 (2023) 61–69
https://doi.org/10.1016/j.coms.2022.06.004
1042-3699/23/© 2022 Elsevier Inc. All rights reserved.

of the craniofacial complex, after which mock-model surgeries are performed on these dental casts. Surgical wafers corresponding to the interim and final occlusions based on the model surgery are fabricated and brought to the operating theater, wherein the surgical repositioning of the first jaw (be it the maxilla or mandible) is determined by an interim occlusion in relation to the second, unoperated jaw, guided by these prefabricated surgical wafers (and an assumed reproducible centric relation of the mandible, in the case that the maxilla is the first operated jaw). The surgical movement of the second jaw would then follow the new position of the first jaw and the final occlusion, guided by the final surgical wafer.

Limitations of Conventional Approach

Several potential limitations are associated with the conventional approach to orthognathic surgery. These limitations arise in various steps during the surgical planning phase that translates to errors intraoperatively. Inaccuracies can occur when assessing the severity of dentofacial deformity by clinical and radiographic assessment, replicating the jaw relationship by facebow transfer and dental casts, errors in model surgery, and errors in the surgical wafers.

Errors in clinical and radiographic assessment
Decisions on surgical movement in conventional orthognathic surgical planning rely on a clinical and radiographic assessment of the patient. Although assessment in the sagittal plane, such as antero-posterior positions of the jaws, as well as the pitch of the maxillomandibular position, is often straightforward, assessment of the jaw and roll of the maxillomandibular position is often difficult. Conventional orthognathic surgical planning often focuses on changes in the sagittal plane based on prediction tracings of lateral cephalograms, whereas the planning for changes in the coronal plane is often overlooked. Moreover, if the shape of the bone—especially in the mandible—is not the same on both sides,[1,2] then this leads to problems because obvious asymmetry may still be present even after the clinician has moved the maxillomandibular complex to the mid-sagittal plane to the best of his/her efforts.

Errors in facebow transfer
It has been shown that inherent errors exist in facebow transfer.[3,4] These errors can occur in the sagittal plane when the horizontal bar of the facebow fails to correspond to the designated horizontal reference plane that is usually the Frankfort horizontal plane. Also, errors can exist in the frontal plane, failing to capture the true clinical canting,

or in the axial plane, inaccurately replicating the true jaw of the dental arch. The possible errors from this method could be inaccuracies in positioning the facebow, mobility of the facebow on the patient, soft tissue hindrance, the flexibility of the metal material of the facebow, and operator errors. These errors in facebow transfer are often compounded, resulting in failure to accurately capture the 3D position of the jaws in relation to the craniofacial complex.

Errors in mounting of dental casts
Imprecisions in facebow-transfer, as well as other inherent errors, such as dimensional changes of gypsum on setting, result in an incorrect 3D position of the mounted maxillary dental cast on the articulator. However, the mounting of the mandibular dental cast utilizes a bite registration in the centric-relation position that is assumed to be reproducible theoretically. However, errors often exist when obtaining a bite registration, because of patients' muscle memory, the accuracy of impression material, and operator technique. This occurs especially in skeletal class II patients who may have a usual bite that is very different from that in centric relation. Moreover, the centric relation position on the operating table may be different than that captured preoperatively, because of positioning as well as the effects of muscle relaxants. Errors in the mounting of dental casts would result in errors in the planning of surgical movements. For example, if the true occlusal canting is not captured by the mounted models, the resulting correction of canting on the patient may be inadequate. Also, in bimaxillary surgery, because the neoposition of the first operated jaw is based on an intermediate wafer in relation to the opposing jaw, errors in the mounting of the opposing jaw would result in an incorrect neoposition of the first operated jaw. This would, in turn, lead to mistakes in the second operated jaw.

VIRTUAL SURGICAL PLANNING: A NEW ERA

The introduction of computed tomography (CT) in the latter part of the 20th century has enhanced medical and surgical treatment in that anatomy can be assessed in 3D. Since then, computer programs have been developed for surgical simulation, in which CT data is converted to digital imaging and communications in medicine (DICOM) files to construct virtual reconstructions of objects, such as the maxillofacial skeleton. Software programs for VSP, such as PROPLAN CMF by Materialize (Leuven, Belgium), allow simulated osteotomy and manipulation of the virtual reconstruction of the craniofacial skeleton. This enables clinicians and technicians to plan for the desired surgical movements while looking at the 3D virtual skull and allows visualization of the feasibility of planned bony movements, such as whether there is any bone contact or bony interferences (**Fig. 1**). Also, when matched with 3D photographic data that is also converted to DICOM files and reconstructed virtually, VSP allows simulation of esthetic results when matched with 3D photography.

Translating Virtual Surgical Planning to Operating Room

VSP is without meaning if the planned movements are not translated to the actual surgery. Without 3D printing technology, such translation is possible by mimicking the digitally planned movement of the stone model surgery on the articulator. Laboratory-made surgical wafers are fabricated based on the stone model surgery as in the

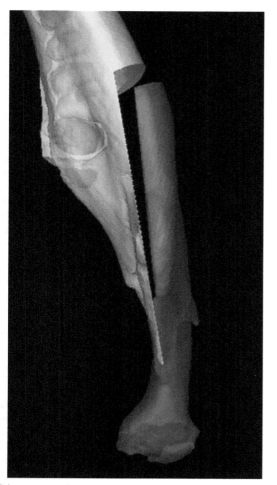

Fig. 1. Virtual surgical planning allows potential bony interferences to be detected.

conventional approach. However, accuracy of this method is poor.

The advent of 3D printing has made an accurate translation from VSP to the operating room possible. Currently, there are two main methods for this translation: (1). 3D printed surgical wafers based on the virtual occlusion and (2). 3D printed personalized cutting guides and PSI. Surgical planning software allows the fabrication of surgical wafers via a 3D printer, using the virtual intermediate and final occlusion that is based on the planned jaw movement. These wafers are brought to the operating room and the surgery is performed as in the conventional approach. However, a major limitation of this approach is that the positioning of the maxilla still depends on the centric relation position of the mandible, in which accuracy may be questionable because of various reasons discussed earlier. Another limitation is that the vertical positioning of the maxilla cannot be translated from the VSP to the patient. A true waferless approach using PSI, in which patient-specific cutting guides and fixation plates are designed based on the virtual surgery simulation, is a more direct approach and has been shown to be superior in accuracy.[5]

TECHNICAL ASPECTS OF PATIENT-SPECIFIC IMPLANTS
Collaboration with Commercial Venders

Orthognathic VSP and fabrication of PSI can be performed in collaboration with commercial vendors. The surgeon sends the patients' CT scans, dental models, or scanned dentition by 3D laser topography and clinical photographs to the engineer. Virtual reconstruction of the craniofacial skeleton by segmentation of CT data and cephalometric analysis can be done by the engineer. The treatment planning for surgical movements and occlusion can be done via video conferencing between the surgeon and the engineer, and the PSI would be designed, printed, and mailed to the surgeon (**Figs. 2 and 3**).

Surgeon-Oriented Approach

Alternatively, VSP and fabrication of PSI can be performed in a surgeon-oriented approach. The main advantages of this approach are that the surgeon would have total control of the whole process and that the time from surgical planning to having the PSI ready for surgery is much faster, because the whole process from planning to product delivery would only take 5–7 days from our experience.[6,7] First of all, the surgeon performs the basic VSP and surgical simulation with virtual planning software. The maxillofacial region of the

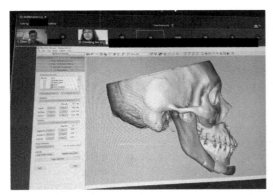

Fig. 2. Video conferencing between surgeons and engineers is widely available for VSP.

patient is scanned with spiral CT with a slice thickness of less than 1.0 mm, or high-resolution cone-beam CT. This imaging data is exported in DICOM format and can then be processed using surgical simulation software. The patient's skull model is virtually reconstructed using the threshold segmentation method that separates the high-density bone tissues from other tissues after choosing a suitable threshold value. For a composite skull model with accurate dentition, stereolithography (STL) files of the dentition obtained by laser topographic scanning are fused with the virtual models of the maxilla and mandible. Osteotomy planes are then designed that correspond to how the cuts would be carried out intraoperatively. The osteotomized bones are then moved to the desired position based on clinical and radiographic findings, as well as determined by measurements on the composite virtual skull model (**Fig. 4**). In practice, the desired final occlusion is often achieved first that can be done based only

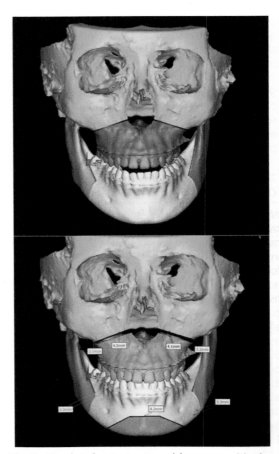

Fig. 4. Simulated osteotomy and bone repositioning by surgeon on a composite virtual skull model using virtual planning software.

on the virtual final occlusion, or matched to the scan of a final occlusion achieved on stone dental casts. After establishing the desired final occlusion, the maxillomandibular complex is then repositioned together as one unit. The movement for the genioplasty segment is performed last. With the incorporation of 3D photography, a prediction of the final esthetic outcome can be performed by the soft tissue simulation function built into the program.

Computer-aided design of patient-specific implants
After surgical simulation, the osteotomized and repositioned virtual composite skull model is then exported as STL files for computer-aided designing of PSI in a 3D-modeling software, such as 3-matic by Materialize (Leuven, Belgium) (**Fig. 5**). The fixation plates are designed first: screw holes are drawn on the bone surface as cylindrical objects, which can be predesigned and

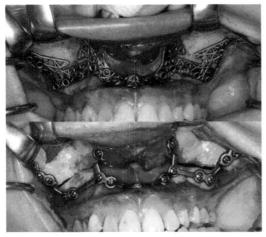

Fig. 3. PSI fabricated by commercial venders used intraoperatively.

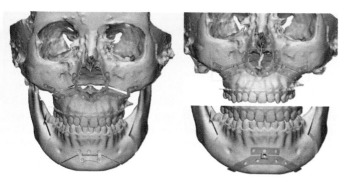

Fig. 5. PSI designed in a surgeon-oriented approach using 3D design software.

saved as templates. Next, the plate is then drawn by connecting the screw holes. Because the connection can only be straight, it can only tolerate very slight curvature on the bone surface. Therefore, if the bone contours between any two screw holes, then the clinician has to put an object between the screw holes to separate the connecting path into two straight lines. For the maxilla, although using separate plates for each side makes it easier to fit onto the bone intraoperatively, a single plate spanning both sides offers better precision in the jaw movement. For the thickness of the plate, a balance has to be achieved in which a plate is made thin while providing adequate mechanical strength. In our experience, the fixation plates are usually between 1 mm – and 1.2 mm thick, with the central connecting portion over the anterior nasal spine made slightly thicker to provide more mechanical strength to minimize the chance of warpage during the manufacturing and transport process.

After designing the fixation plates, the surgical cutting guides are designed using a reverse-engineering technique. The cylindrical objects representing the screw holes and the osteotomized segment of the bone are repositioned together back to the original position of the bone. Now, the screw holes on the stationary and the osteotomized segments of the bone represent the drill holes on the surgical cutting guides. Drill guides can be added by inserting cylindrical objects on top of the drill holes in the same angulation, thus the drill guides serve to guide the angulation of the surgical drill as well as the subsequent placement of the fixation plate. The cutting slots on the surgical guides are designed based on the planned osteotomy plane to allow accurate execution of the planned osteotomy. The cutting slots and drill holes are integrated into the bone-borne surgical guide.

Three-dimensional printing of patient-specific implants

The designed fixation plates and surgical guides are exported to STL format for 3D printing. The fixation plates can be printed with Grade 2 pure titanium using selective laser melting (SLM) technology using specific SLM printers that melt titanium powder into a solid entity using a high-energy laser.[8] After 3D printing, the supporting units are removed, and the titanium plates are polished, cleansed, and sterilized before in vivo implantation. The cutting guides can be 3D-printed in the same way using Grade 2 pure titanium (**Fig. 6**). Alternatively, other biocompatible materials can be used for 3D printing of cutting guides,

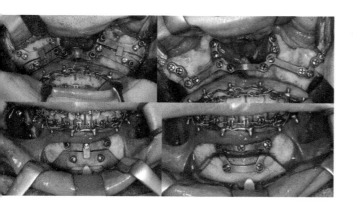

Fig. 6. PSI designed in a surgeon-oriented approach being used intraoperatively.

such as MED610 Resin (Stratasys Ltd., United States) that is printed using fused deposition modeling technology and is resistant to high-temperature autoclaving. Although resin is a more of an economical option, the authors prefer titanium cutting guides. First of all, titanium is a thinner material that makes it easier to fit onto the bone surface intraoperatively. Moreover, there is a higher chance for a resin surgical guide to breaking, either intraoperatively or during the transport process.

ACCURACY OF PATIENT-SPECIFIC IMPLANTS FOR ORTHOGNATHIC SURGERY

The main reason for advancing from the conventional method to the use of PSI for osteosynthesis in orthognathic surgery is the expected benefit of increased accuracy that (supposedly) matches the plan. The use of 3D-printed PSI for other surgical conditions is also blooming.[9] In orthopedic surgery, the applications in hip and knee arthroplasties and bone fracture fixation have proved to give good stability and alignment.[10–12] In the craniomaxillofacial region, the accuracies of PSI for cranioplasty, orbital floor fracture, jaw reconstruction, and orthognathic surgery were studied extensively.[13–16] Various clinical conditions have different expectations and requirements on the accuracies of the applications. In orthognathic surgery, the position of the jaw bones determines the facial profile and symmetry as well as the dental occlusion that are essential for good facial esthetic and masticatory function. In contrast to the PSI used in cranioplasty and orbital floor reconstruction that the implants replace the original structure to repair a defect, orthognathic PSI aims to orientate and fixate a mobilized jaw bone to a new position that is planned preoperatively. The assessment of the accuracy of orthognathic PSI, therefore, is on the jaw position rather than the PSI. The requirement to achieve high accuracy in orthognathic surgery PSI is therefore technically demanding.

The accuracy of the orthognathic surgery by PSI is by comparing the postoperative jaw position against the planned model in the computer virtual planning. A systematic review concluded that a linear deviation within 2 mm for all three axes, and an angular deviation within 2.7° in pitch, roll, or jaw were considered to be accurate in a virtually planned orthognathic surgery that is positioned with an occlusal wafer.[17] Le Fort I osteotomy performed by PSI uses a waferless approach to reposition and fix the maxilla. Heufelder and colleagues[18] reported the use of a commercially available PSI system for single-piece Le Fort I

osteotomies with a median linear deviation of 0.39 mm from the virtual planning. The group also reported that the antero-posterior dimension deviated more when compared with lateral or vertical dimensions.[18] Suojanen and colleagues[19] reported in a larger case series with 3D-printed plastic surgical guides and titanium PSI that 31 out of 32 cases had a good fit of the PSI and were able to achieve the planned movement. Our group has performed a thorough assessment of the accuracy using a self-designed titanium surgical guide and PSI. In our study, we found the linear deviation in the x, y, and z axes ranged from 0.72 mm to 0.75 mm, and the deviations in the principal axes of pitch, roll, and jaw were 1.40°, 0.90°, and 0.60°, respectively.[20] These findings indicate that in general waferless Le Fort I osteotomy is highly accurate and appears to be superior to those performed with wafer positioning that is reported in the literature. However, among the three principal axes, the pitch was found to be relatively less accurate when compared with the roll and jaw planes. We consider that the pitch is relatively less controlled because of the further distance from the PSI fixation and allows more deviation in the plane. Of note, a larger deviation in the pitch plane would not affect symmetry because it is determined by the roll and jaw planes. Genioplasty using PSI is also proved to be highly accurate. Several studies showed the linear deviation of the genioplasty was within 0.7 mm.[21,22] A case series of our group to assess the accuracy of the self-designed genioplasty PSI was found to be 0.19 mm.[6] These findings prove that the resulting bone repositioning using PSI highly matches that of the virtual planning in orthognathic procedures. The accurate positioning allows orthognathic surgeons to execute the plan with a clinically insignificant discrepancy.

SOLUTION FOR ALL PROBLEMS? PROS AND CONS OF PATIENT-SPECIFIC IMPLANTS

We have discussed the major advantage of using PSI in orthognathic procedures is that its high accuracy. The waferless approach in Le Fort I osteotomy avoids the reliance on opposing occlusion as well as the TMJ rotation that could be sources of error in positioning the maxilla.[18] In cases with significant asymmetry, the axes of movement of the TMJ for mouth opening and closing could be a curvilinear path. Such motion could not be mimicked by articulators or virtual planning that leads to unrecognized error when using a wafer approach to position the maxillary segment. With PSI, the maxilla can be positioned irrespective of the opposing mandible or the TMJ rotational

A
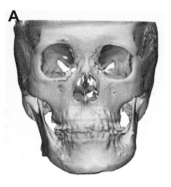

B
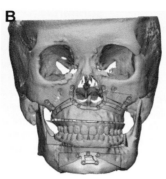

Fig. 7. Patients with asymmetry may benefit from more accurate positioning of the maxilla through a waferless PSI approach irrespective of the opposing mandible or the TMJ rotational path. (*A*) Preoperative; (*B*) planned waferless Le Fort I osteotomy and genioplasty with PSI application.

path (**Fig. 7**). In addition, the vertical dimension is a variable that is adjustable intraoperatively when using wafers to position the maxillary segment. In contrast, PSI determines the vertical dimension through the pre-existing screw holes according to the virtual planning. PSI is particularly helpful in performing genioplasty. The osteosynthesis of conventional genioplasty mostly relies on free-hand positioning and fixation of the chin segment with plates and/or screws that in fact involves intraoperative eye-balling and possibly an artistic sense of the chief surgeon to achieve an esthetic result with good symmetry.[23] Intraoperative trial and error is often required, and the prefabricated genioplasty fixation plates may not fit perfectly onto the bony architecture of the chin segment. With the use of PSI, the movement and symmetry of the genioplasty follow the predetermined plan. The time spent on the procedure is also greatly reduced. The surgeons can follow the surgical guide and screw holes to perform a fast yet accurate genioplasty procedure with confidence.

Knowing the benefits, it is important to understand the limitations of PSI for orthognathic surgery. The following limitations/disadvantages should be considered: (1) high cost; (2) turnaround time; (3) possibility of ill-fitting surgical guide or PSI; (4) inability to perform intraoperative adjustment; and (5) bony interferences are not easily noticeable. It is known that various commercially available PSI charge much more than prefabricated osteosynthetic material of the same company. The costs normally include a consultation session with the medical engineer, the design and the fabrication of the surgical guide and PSI, and the delivery of the product. It is understood that 3D-printed medical grade material, in particular printed metal, and the new technology justify a higher cost. Yet, it is a practical consideration that the extra costs of orthognathic surgery may affect the choice of the osteosynthesis method.[24] The concept of surgeon-designed PSI may help

to reduce the costs; however, the regulations of many countries only allow approved commercial implant products for surgical use.[6] For the turnaround time, it was reported a range of 15 days–42 days from planning to product delivery would be required depending on the companies' support and the location of the orthognathic center[6,18,24] that is longer than that of a conventional or virtually planned wafer-guided orthognathic procedure.

Occasionally, the surgical guide or PSI is found to be ill-fitting on the bony architecture during the surgery. It could be a production error or distortion of the printed titanium framework, or more frequently it could be the irregularities of thin bone or teeth roots on the surface of the maxilla that cause interferences to the adaption of the surgical guide or PSI (**Fig. 8**). In our center, an intermediate wafer is always prepared as a contingency plan in case the printed framework is found to be ill-fitting, although the occurrence is rare. Moreover, the beauty of the accuracy of PSI could also be a disadvantage in case the intraoperative adjustment is required, which would not be feasible for PSI cases. It requires more consideration of the soft tissue changes as a result of the surgical movement to ensure the plan need not be

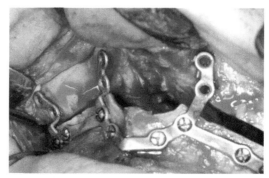

Fig. 8. Ill-fitting of PSI may occur as a consequence of framework distortion or bony interference.

adjusted intraoperatively for a good esthetic outcome. Furthermore, the use of a 3D-printed surgical guide and PSI still requires an understanding of the surgical movement and anatomy. Minute bony interferences may not be easily detected but could cause ill-fitting of the PSI and the jaw segment. From our experience, it is particularly challenging for an impaction and setback movement of the Le Fort I osteotomy, where the posterior and superior bony interferences at the pterygoid plates are difficult to be noticed but yet hinder a passive fitting of the PSI. Extra effort to remove all interferences is often required to achieve the planned movements. These limitations need to be acknowledged in the decision of applying PSI for orthognathic surgery.

ORTHOGNATHIC PATIENT-SPECIFIC IMPLANTS: WHERE DOES THE FUTURE LIE?

The rapid development of virtual planning and 3D printing in the recent decade has boosted the increasing popularity of the use of PSI for orthognathic surgery. The high accuracy and minimal complications are attractive to most orthognathic centers for routine application.[6] The high cost of PSI is by far the biggest hurdle to surgeons and patients, in particular to those in lower socioeconomic groups and developing countries. It is expected the costs will lower in the future when more companies are providing the service. With the development of open-source computer planning and PSI design software programs, surgeons/medical technicians can plan and design PSI in their offices, which can then be exported for production. Some centers have pioneered in this field of designing PSI in-house.[6,24] Currently, the cost of 3D printers to print medical-grade titanium PSI is still high and not easily accessible. There is a need to produce low-cost hospital-based metal printers when the technology is more mature. Various printable materials are being tested for the purpose of osteosynthesis. Tantalum and magnesium alloys are showing promising results to replace titanium for osteosynthesis.[25] Other nonmetallic materials may also serve a similar purpose but biocompatibility and biomechanical studies are required to prove the feasibility.[26] In principle, degradable biomaterials with the incorporation of growth factors to induce bone formation could also be printed and used for bone fixation.[27,28] A surge of discoveries of 3D-printed osteosynthetic material for clinical use is expected in the coming years. It is foreseeable that the routine use of PSI for various surgical conditions, including orthognathic surgery, could be the standard-of-care in the near future.

SUMMARY

Owing to the introduction of 3D medical imaging, the emergence of VSP software, and 3D printing technology, we have seen a rapid rise in the development of computer-aided surgery and PSI in recent years. These new advances have circumvented the limitations of the conventional approach, such as shortcomings of 2D-based assessment, errors in facebow transfer, reliance on the TMJ rotational path in positioning the maxilla, and intraoperative "guesstimate" of the vertical maxillary position. PSI has the benefits of high accuracy and having the ability to reproduce the bony movements from the virtual plan to the patient that can be especially useful in challenging cases, such as those cases with significant asymmetry. Although it is without a doubt that the popularity of PSI will continue to increase in the future, as the technology becomes more accessible and the cost of 3D printing becomes lower, there will still be times when the hardware fails to fit or produce the desired repositioning, or when intraoperative alterations of the planned movements are desired. Therefore, it is still important for young surgeons to go through training in the conventional approach before advancing to orthognathic surgery with PSI.

CLINICS CARE POINTS

- There are limitations of wafer-based approach of orthognathic surgery.
- Waferless approach of orthognathic surgery by patient-specific implant reduces the surgical errors and inaccuracies.

REFERENCES

1. Leung MY, Leung YY. Three-dimensional evaluation of mandibular asymmetry: a new classification and three-dimensional cephalometric analysis. Int J Oral Maxillofac Surg 2018;47(8):1043–51.
2. Yeung AWK, Wong NSM, Li DTS, et al. Is there a difference between the thicknesses of the rami in mandibular asymmetry? Int J Oral Maxillofac Surg 2021;50(6):791–7.
3. Quast A, Santander P, Witt D, et al. Traditional facebow transfer versus three-dimensional virtual reconstruction in orthognathic surgery. Int J Oral Maxillofac Surg 2019;48(3):347–54.
4. Zizelmann C, Hammer B, Gellrich NC, et al. An evaluation of face-bow transfer for the planning of

orthognathic surgery. J Oral Maxillofac Surg 2012; 70(8):1944–50.

5. Li B, Wei H, Jiang T, et al. Randomized Clinical Trial of the Accuracy of Patient-Specific Implants versus CAD/CAM Splints in Orthognathic Surgery. Plast Reconstr Surg 2021;148(5):1101–10.

6. Au SW, Li DTS, Su YX, et al. Accuracy of Self-designed 3D-Printed Patient-Specific Surgical Guides and Fixation Plates for Advancement Genioplasty<<<<<. Int J Comput Dent 2022;0(0):0.

7. Yang WF, Zhang CY, Choi WS, et al. A novel 'surgeon-dominated' approach to the design of 3D-printed patient-specific surgical plates in mandibular reconstruction: a proof-of-concept study. Int J Oral Maxillofac Surg 2020;49(1):13–21.

8. Attar H, Calin M, Zhang LC, et al. Manufacture by selective laser melting and mechanical behavior of commercially pure titanium. Mater Sci Eng A 2014; 593:170–7.

9. Haglin JM, Eltorai AE, Gil JA, et al. Patient-Specific Orthopaedic Implants. Orthop Surg 2016;8(4): 417–24.

10. Cheng T, Zhao S, Peng X, et al. Does computer-assisted surgery improve postoperative leg alignment and implant positioning following total knee arthroplasty? A meta-analysis of randomized controlled trials? Knee Surg Sports Traumatol Arthrosc 2012;20(7):1307–22.

11. Small T, Krebs V, Molloy R, et al. Comparison of acetabular shell position using patient specific instruments vs. standard surgical instruments: a randomized clinical trial. J Arthroplasty 2014;29(5): 1030–7.

12. Schemitsch EH, Richards RR. The effect of malunion on functional outcome after plate fixation of fractures of both bones of the forearm in adults. J Bone Joint Surg Am 1992;74(7):1068–78.

13. van de Vijfeijken S, Schreurs R, Dubois L, et al. The use of cranial resection templates with 3D virtual planning and PEEK patient-specific implants: A 3 year follow-up. J Craniomaxillofac Surg 2019;47(4): 542–7.

14. Gander T, Essig H, Metzler P, et al. Patient specific implants (PSI) in reconstruction of orbital floor and wall fractures. J Craniomaxillofac Surg 2015;43(1): 126–30.

15. Yang WF, Choi WS, Leung YY, et al. Three-dimensional printing of patient-specific surgical plates in head and neck reconstruction: A prospective pilot study. Oral Oncol 2018;78:31–6.

16. Rückschloß T, Ristow O, Müller M, et al. Accuracy of patient-specific implants and additive-manufactured surgical splints in orthognathic surgery - A three-dimensional retrospective study. J Craniomaxillofac Surg 2019;47(6):847–53.

17. Alkhayer A, Piffkó J, Lippold C, et al. Accuracy of virtual planning in orthognathic surgery: a systematic review. Head Face Med 2020;16(1):34.

18. Heufelder M, Wilde F, Pietzka S, et al. Clinical accuracy of waferless maxillary positioning using customized surgical guides and patient specific osteosynthesis in bimaxillary orthognathic surgery. J Craniomaxillofac Surg 2017;45(9):1578–85.

19. Suojanen J, Leikola J, Stoor P. The use of patient-specific implants in orthognathic surgery: A series of 32 maxillary osteotomy patients. J Craniomaxillofac Surg 2016;44(12):1913–6.

20. Leung YY, Leung JKC, Li ATC et al. Accuracy and Safety of In-House Surgeon-Designed Three-Dimensional Printed Patient Specific Implants for Wafer-less Le Fort I Osteotomy. Hong Kong International Dental Expo And Symposium; December 10–12, 2021; Hong Kong 2021.

21. Rückschloß T, Ristow O, Kühle R, et al. Accuracy of laser-melted patient-specific implants in genioplasty - A three-dimensional retrospective study. J Craniomaxillofac Surg 2020;48(7):653–60.

22. Li B, Wang S, Wei H, et al. The use of patient-specific implants in genioplasty and its clinical accuracy: a preliminary study. Int J Oral Maxillofac Surg 2020;49(4):461–5.

23. Li B, Wei H, Zeng F, et al. Application of A Novel Three-dimensional Printing Genioplasty Template System and Its Clinical Validation: A Control Study. Sci Rep 2017;7(1):5431.

24. Goodson AMC, Parmar S, Ganesh S, et al. Printed titanium implants in UK craniomaxillofacial surgery. Part II: perceived performance (outcomes, logistics, and costs). Br J Oral Maxillofac Surg 2021;59(3): 320–8.

25. Ma L, Cheng S, Ji X, et al. Immobilizing magnesium ions on 3D printed porous tantalum scaffolds with polydopamine for improved vascularization and osteogenesis. Mater Sci Eng C Mater Biol Appl 2020; 117:111303.

26. Kabiri A, Liaghat G, Alavi F, et al. A comparative study of 3D printing and heat-compressing methods for manufacturing the thermoplastic composite bone fixation plate: Design, characterization, and in vitro biomechanical experimentation. Proc Inst Mech Eng H 2021;235(12):1439–52.

27. MacLeod A, Patterson M, MacTear K, et al. 3D printed locking osteosynthesis screw threads have comparable strength to machined or hand-tapped screw threads. J Orthop Res 2020;38(7):1559–65.

28. Esmaeili S, Akbari Aghdam H, Motififard M, et al. A porous polymeric-hydroxyapatite scaffold used for femur fractures treatment: fabrication, analysis, and simulation. Eur J Orthop Surg Traumatol 2020; 30(1):123–31.

Surgery First and Surgery Early Treatment Approach in Orthognathic Surgery

Gabriele A. Millesi, MD, DMD[a],*, Matthias Zimmermann, MD, DMD[a],
Maija Eltz, MD, DMD[b]

KEYWORDS

- Orthognathic surgery • Treatment protocol • Surgery first approach • Surgery early approach
- Digital planning

KEY POINTS

- Surgery First approach or Surgery Early approach should be included in the consideration of orthognathic surgery planning with the input from both the surgeon and the orthodontist.
- Surgery First approach allows an immediate correction of the skeletal discrepancies of the patients and shortens the overall treatment time.
- Surgery Early approach may help to eliminate some unfavorable factors of Surgery First approach, such as postoperative instability or occlusal disharmony (eg, insufficient overbite, such as compromised inter-canine width).

HISTORICAL BACKGROUND

At the beginning of orthognathic surgery in the 1960s, surgeons, independent of their background, whether plastic or oral maxillofacial surgeons, were forced to do the Surgery First approach when they wanted to correct a skeletal deformity because there was no efficient orthodontic treatment available at that time. The goal of the treatment plan was mainly driven by correcting the skeletal deformity, harmonizing the skeleton, and achieving the best possible jaw relation, but accepting minor discrepancies of the Angle classes, misalignments, or crossbites of the dental arches. The consequence was a deficit of perfect functional rehabilitation and in the long term, a lack of predictability and stability of the achieved surgical results.

It was in the 1980s with William Bell[1,2] that a paradigm shift in orthognathic surgery was introduced. With the rapid development of orthodontic appliances and improvement of techniques, it became obvious that any preoperative removal of dental obstacles in the occlusion was advantageous for the surgeon in two ways. A stable interdigitation was created in the preoperative setup, according to the aligned dental arches, which signaled stability of the postoperative results, and the final occlusion became the center of imagination and the face was built around by osteotomizing the jaws. In fact, this is a perfect concept for the surgeon, the orthodontist, and the patient.

INTRODUCTION

The concept of preoperative orthodontics followed by surgery, called the Orthodontics First approach, was the state-of-the-art for nearly half a century and still is routinely done, especially in the Anglo-American and the Western world.

As described by J.W. Choi in his book titled, *The Surgery–First Orthognathic Approach* in 2002, a new treatment protocol was published by a Korean study group in the *Korean Journal of Clinical Orthodontics* on a new treatment concept called "Functional Orthognathic Surgery."[3] There are some controversies on the founders of the

[a] Department of Oral and Maxillofacial Surgery, Medical University Vienna, Waehringerguertel 18-20, Vienna 1090, Austria; [b] Dr. Maija Eltz Institut für Kieferorthopädie, Dorotheergasse 7/5, Vienna 1010, Austria
* Corresponding author.
E-mail address: gabriele.millesi@meduniwien.ac.at

Oral Maxillofacial Surg Clin N Am 35 (2023) 71–82
https://doi.org/10.1016/j.coms.2022.06.010
1042-3699/23/© 2022 Elsevier Inc. All rights reserved.

Surgery First approach because of different definitions of the approach, and mode of concomitant orthodontic treatment pre-op or primarily post-op. The new concept of orthognathic surgery was well and fast taken and put in place especially in Korea, Japan and, Taiwan with minor individualizations.[4–7]

Societies change, and lifestyles and expectations of our patients change, too. Esthetic improvements have moved to the foreground and visible results are expected within a short time. Especially in the Asian world, this was strongly boosted by the mass media but because we are living in a global environment with online connections, this trend was quickly picked up internationally. And action provokes a reaction, especially in the western hemisphere any preoperative orthodontic treatment was expanded up to two years which created an unacceptable and unfavorable overall long treatment time for the patients.

Any Surgery First or Surgery Early treatment approach includes the advantage of reduced treatment time. We know from the previous publications[8] that in the conventional Orthodontics First approach, the preoperative treatment time is prolonged and that the overall treatment period in bimaxillary cases can last about 18–28 months.[9] In contrast, in the Surgery First approach, the overall treatment time is reduced to about 38 weeks on average as published by Hernández-Alfaro and colleagues,[10] which corresponds with our own observation. The difference between the two treatment options is the number of appointments with the orthodontists. In the Surgery First approach cases that require extractions combined with maxillary segmentations, the postoperative orthodontic treatment times may be slightly prolonged when compared to single-piece nonextraction cases.[11]

THE ADVANTAGE OF SURGERY FIRST

There is an additional reason why the Surgery First protocol was well taken in the Asian region. The predominant skeletal deformity in the Asian region is skeletal Class III, with protrusive mandible and retrusive maxilla. Baik and colleagues[12] reported the percentage of Korean patients whose Class III relationship was primarily a result of mandibular prognathism (48%), which is more than twice as high as the corresponding number for American Class III surgical patients (19%), somewhat higher than in Chinese (39%), and similar to the percentage of Japanese patients (50%). In the traditional Orthodontics First concept, the orthodontist decompensates the lower incisors of the patients with Class III deformities, which is a procedure

that has to be done slowly and cautiously to avoid buccal recessions. The aim of the dental alignment was to allow the surgeon to create a correct overbite/overjet by the time of the surgery. For the patient, however, especially in Skeletal Class III patients (**Fig. 1**), this period of decompensation is extremely unfavorable functionally and esthetically, which aggravates the unpleasant profile. Surgery First approach allows immediate correction of the deformity and is executed by creating a Class II relationship with an increased overjet intraoperatively for later proclination of the incisors (**Fig. 2**). Besides, there are observations that these exaggerated protrusive movements of the lower incisors during decompensation are prone to relapse because of the mild muscular relapse of the surgical setback of the protrusive mandible.[13]

Questionnaire studies[14] explored the patient's perception of the combined orthognathic/orthodontic treatment and showed that the period of the orthodontic treatment was the most uncomfortable of the whole treatment. Therefore, shortening of orthodontics time is welcomed.

Rapid acceleratory phenomenon (RAP) is one of the explanations why the postsurgical orthodontic treatment is more effective and faster. The accelerated orthodontic movement after surgery was not new, which was demonstrated after corticotomies as described by Kole.[15] Wilcko and colleagues[16] also demonstrated the effect by performing corticotomies in combination with alveolar buccal augmentation in the lower frontal incisors. In a literature review, Frost further explained the RAP and the bone healing process.[17] Le Fort I osteotomy or the sagittal split osteotomy alone can act as a booster of the RAP, which is also confirmed in an animal study by Yuan and colleagues.[18] The increased tooth mobility and highly effective orthodontic treatment are mirrored in the increased levels of serum alkaline phosphatase and the C-terminal telopeptide of type I collagen, corresponding to the altered and stimulated bone metabolism due to surgery.[19] By measuring the serum levels of these two predictors, the time frame of the advantage of the RAP can be estimated. This window of accelerated tooth movement is observed up to 3–4 months after surgery and therefore early postoperative start of orthodontic treatment is mandatory to take advantage of the biomechanics of bone healing. Corticotomies in the buccal area of the lower incisors can be seen not only as an attempt to stimulate the RAP, but also to ease the additional mechanical tooth movement to align the dental arches.[20]

Attention is also brought to the permanent soft tissue resistance of lip pressure or tongue thrust

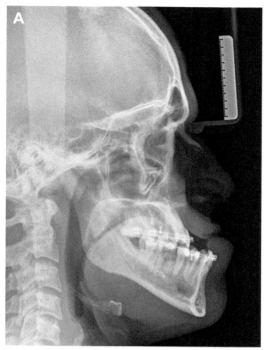

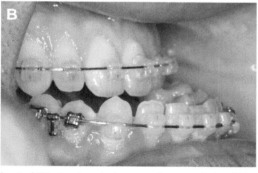

Fig. 1. (*A*) Lateral cephalogram of severe skeletal Class III treated with Orthodontic First approach after 1.5 years of preoperative orthodontic decompensation. (*B*). Intraoral view of severe skeletal Class III treated with Orthodontic First approach after 1.5 years of preoperative orthodontic decompensation.

and dysfunction, especially in Class III skeletal deformity and open bite cases during the preoperative orthodontic period in Orthodontics First approach. A rapid skeletal correction and harmonization of the dysfunctional situations ease any postoperative orthodontic treatment by overcoming the muscle tensions.

The Selection of Patients for Surgery First Treatment Protocol

A successful outcome of orthognathic surgery based on a Surgery First concept depends

primarily on the selection of the appropriate patient as well as a suitable orthodontist partner (**Fig. 3**). The orthodontist has to be familiar with the Surgery First concept, who is willing to take over after surgery, and capable to correct the postsurgical occlusion to finish the case. Therefore, it is of uttermost importance that the surgical treatment plan is discussed and agreed upon with the orthodontist. In general, the orthodontist comes up with a piggyback occlusal setup that is used for orientation in the surgical concept (**Fig. 4**). There are several considerations for postoperative occlusion. First of all, it is important to consider if a stable occlusion is achievable intraoperatively without preoperative orthodontics (**Fig. 5**). Sharma and colleagues[21] suggested the ideal case for the Surgery First approach is a patient with well-aligned dental arches and minimal crowding. This requires no segmentation of the osteotomies, due to no transversal discrepancies and no need for extractions to flatten any exaggerated Curves of Spee. Many of these cases are patients who already had orthodontic treatment in their teens when no regard was taken for any forthcoming skeletal deformity at the time of adulthood. When they grow up, the genetically determined skeletal deformity appears and makes an additional correction of the malocclusion necessary. It is understandable that these patients who already had orthodontic therapy for years in their adolescence are not willing to start orthodontics again for the orthognathic surgery preparation at the end of growth. Many would prefer an accelerated, efficient treatment path as seen in the Surgery First approach. From a surgeon's perspective, the surgical procedures per se are of no difference to that of a conventional Orthodontics First approach. These patients are excellent candidates as a starting point for the surgeon and the orthodontist who are inexperienced in the Surgery First approach. Another challenge of the Surgery First approach is the decision between bimaxillary and single jaw procedures. In contrast to the conventional Orthodontic First approach, Surgery First approach lacks the chance to reassess the treatment plan for a second time and has to make a correct decision at the beginning of the orthognathic treatment planning. Falter and colleagues[22] reported a 13.5% chance that the executed treatment protocol will differ from the originally designed one, therefore any surgical planning in the Surgery First approach must be well weighted to avoid any unnecessary secondary procedures. The third group, as presented in **Fig. 3**, is a cohort with extended dental and skeletal deformities, patients with severe crowding, exaggerated Curves of Spee, and/or

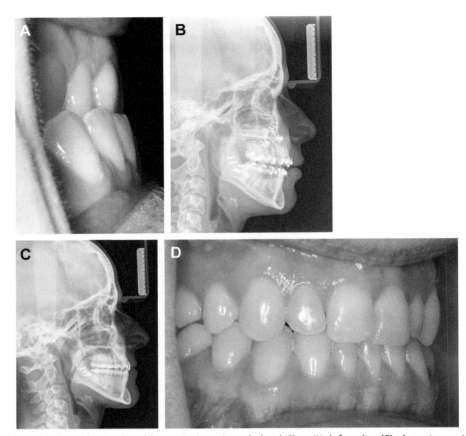

Fig. 2. (*A*) Lateral view of retroclined lower incisors in a skeletal Class III deformity. (*B*). A postoperative lateral cephalogram showing the planned Class II occlusion to create an overjet to allow proclination lower incisors post-surgically in Surgery First approach. (*C*). Lateral cephalogram at postoperative one year. (*D*). Final occlusion at postoperative one year.

transversal discrepancies (**Fig. 6**). Treating these patients requires a lot more considerations in the surgical planning, with a need for more surgical expertise and experience that segmental osteotomies combined with extractions may be required because the complex surgery is needed to take over any orthodontic preoperative alignment (**Fig. 7**). Besides, it is obligatory that the patient is fully informed about the strategy of the Surgery First approach in comparison to the prolonged and more conservative procedure of the Orthodontics First approach. A signed consent form of the patient is required, highlighting that the patient was informed about different treatment options.[23] The explanation also has to include that the Surgery First approach is combined with the expected compliance of the patient for the postoperative frequent orthodontic appointments. Short control intervals with the surgeon and the orthodontist are essential postoperatively because teeth movements are accelerated because of the RAP (**Fig. 8**).

Surgery First Approach in Skeletal Class III Deformity

The correction of a skeletal Class III deformity is the predominant indication for Surgery First approach because any preoperative orthodontic treatment for decompensation means additional psychological and functional pressure on the patient. Standard surgical planning is performed by three-dimensional (3D) virtual planning nowadays.[24] This includes a Cone Beam Computer Tomography (CBCT) with a defined occlusion by a splint, an intraoral scan, and standardized photos. The CBCT DICOM (Digital Imaging and Communications in Medicine) data of the skeletal bone and the STL (Standard Triangle Language) file of the occlusion are fused, with the natural head position transferred via radiopaque markers and laser beam into the CBCT. The surgical planning can then be processed in a software program. Any planning in the Surgery First approach starts with

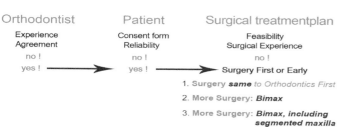

Flowchart

Patients Selection for Surgery First

Orthodontist | Patient | Surgical treatmentplan

Experience | Consent form | Feasibility
Agreement | Reliability | Surgical Experience
no ! | no ! | no !
yes ! ⟶ | yes ! ⟶ | Surgery First or Early

1. Surgery *same* to Orthodontics First
2. More Surgery: *Bimax*
3. More Surgery: *Bimax, including segmented maxilla*

Fig. 3. Flowchart of criteria of selection for Surgery First patients: three pillars to rely on: the orthodontist, the patient, and surgical treatment plan, which can be subdivided into another three approaches: (1) Surgery as in case of Orthodontic First approach, (2) bimaxillary surgery to avoid any additional secondary surgical procedure, and (3) more aggressive surgery because any optional preoperative orthodontic alignment has to be done surgically.

the definition of the position, the angulation, and the expected show of the upper incisors. If there is hardly any crowding and quite nicely aligned dental arches, but a retrusive maxilla and protrusive mandible, the necessary movements of the jaws do not differ from the conventional Orthodontics First approach but only the amount of sagittal movement and clockwise rotation. In the Surgery First approach, one has to create an exaggerated Class II (see **Fig. 2**B) overjet for postoperative orthodontic proclination of the lower incisors. To keep control over this intermediate occlusion and the mandible which is relatively unstable, there are different approaches. As described by Nagasaka and colleagues and Sugawara and

colleagues,[4,5] it is possible to stabilize the upper and lower molar relation by a wafer sparing the incisors during this period, or by temporary anchorage devices and elastics. Especially in cases of open bite deformities with extreme vertical growth patterns and vertical excess in the molar area, the Surgery First approach has its advantages. Any preoperative orthodontic leveling of the dental arches in those deformities may result in some mild degree of compensation of the original skeletal deformity either by extrusion of the frontal teeth or intrusion and tilting of the molars. The result is a risk of instability and relapse after surgery because the surgical plan is not on the original degree of the skeletal deformity but on the

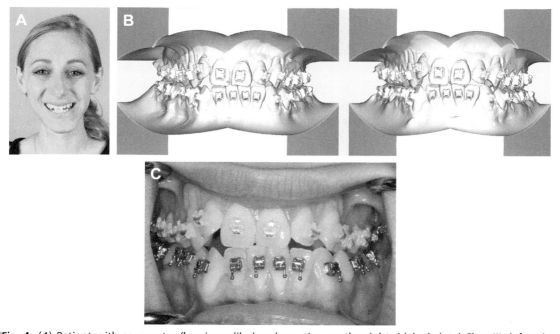

Fig. 4. (*A*) Patient with asymmetry (hemimandibular elongation on the right side), skeletal Class III deformity, compensatory maxillary canting on the right side. (*B*). Simulated preoperative piggyback occlusion designed by the orthodontist. (*C*). Preoperative occlusion with brackets bonded before surgery.

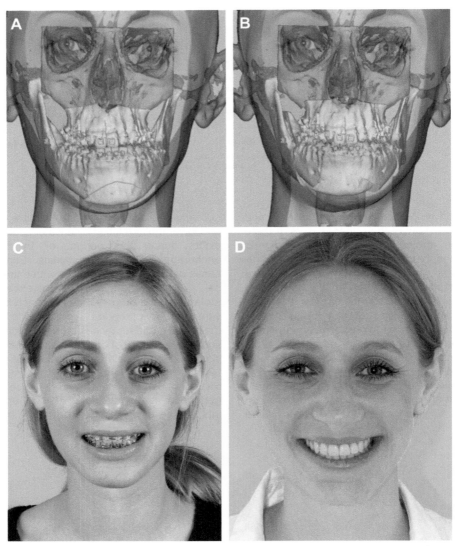

Fig. 5. (*A*) Preoperative situation. (*B*). 3D virtual planning of the bimaxillary surgery and genioplasty, with asymmetric impaction of the maxilla by Le Fort I osteotomy and differential mandibular setback by bilateral sagittal split osteotomies. (*C*). Result 3 months after Surgery First approach correction. (*D*). Final outcome, with an overall treatment of 8 months.

actual presenting, post-orthodontic situation. Epker and Fish[25] supported the Surgery First approach with this argument, even against the general established trend of the Orthodontics First approach in the 1980s. In times of digital planning, the surgeon now has better visualization and control of the desired occlusion in the preoperative setup by simulating segmentations and leveling of the extended Curve of Spee. Choi and colleagues[26]. commented in their book titled, *The Surgery-First Orthognathic Approach* in the chapter titled, "SFA controversies," that excessively extruded upper second molars, severe crowding of the upper anterior incisors, and disharmony between upper and lower inter-canine widths would be a contraindication for the Surgery First approach. We do agree that these circumstances need meticulous consideration to be treated successfully and safely. Turvey and colleagues[27] also proposed that vertical segmentation of the osteotomy requires an interdental bony bridge up to 5 mm to avoid injury to the adjacent roots. In case of the Surgery First approach, no presurgical inter-radicular gap was created orthodontically. Therefore, an estimation of the feasibility must be evaluated digitally and visualization of the

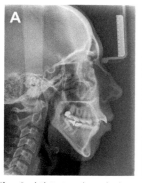
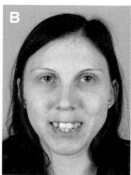
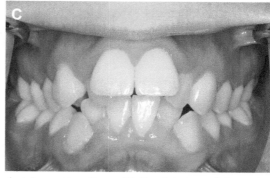

Fig. 6. (A) Lateral cephalogram of a patient with dolichofacial growth pattern. (B). Frontal view of the patient with dolichofacial growth pattern. (C). Occlusion with severe crowding.

angulation of the adjacent roots is mandatory. In the case of a compressed maxilla, premolar extractions and segmentation through the extraction socket are an option, which can be used as a rotation point between the anterior and posterior segments to change the angulations as well as widen the maxilla in the transverse dimension. If the inter-canine distance is compromised and the radius of the anterior segment is small, then it is impossible to create a stable postoperative overbite. This is a severe problem and contraindication for a Surgery First approaches (**Fig. 9**A) unless additional midline segmentation between the two incisors is performed (**Fig. 9**B). It is technically feasible but may increase the risk of poor vascularity of the segments and the interdental papilla. This decision of executing a four-piece segmentation of the dental arch strongly depends on the overall movement of the maxilla, the amount of expansion of the segments, the periodontal health of the gingiva, and whether the patient is a smoker or not. To stay on the safe side, we advocate managing those cases with insufficient inter-canine width in a Surgery Early approach as discussed in the following sections. DICODICOM

Surgery First Approach in Skeletal Class II Deformity

Skeletal Class II division 2 deformity is a limitation to performing osteotomies by a Surgery First approach. In these cases, the upper dental arch has to be aligned first, followed by a bilateral sagittal split osteotomy to advance the mandible, which allows the establishment of a desired over-bite and overjet based on a postoperative tripod occlusion. To close the vertical open bite in the molar and premolar areas, the orthodontist will take advantage of anchor screws or plates if there is an exaggerated Curve of Spee in place in the lower dental arch, which avoids an undesired extrusion of the upper molars and premolars.

When and Why Altering the Surgery First Protocol to Surgery Early Approach?

Recent 3D virtual planning including a digital setup of the occlusion and customized orthodontic wires has created new possibilities for early surgery in cases that were originally considered as a contra-indication for the Surgery First approach. These are primarily cases where aggressive leveling and alignment of the dental arches are necessary

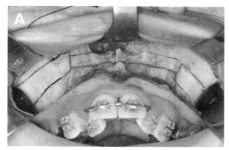
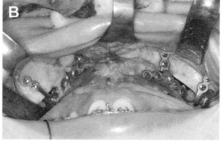

Fig. 7. (A) Intraoperative photos showing the designed osteotomies for impaction and vertical segmentation via extraction socket of premolars. (B). Osteosynthesis of the segmented maxilla.

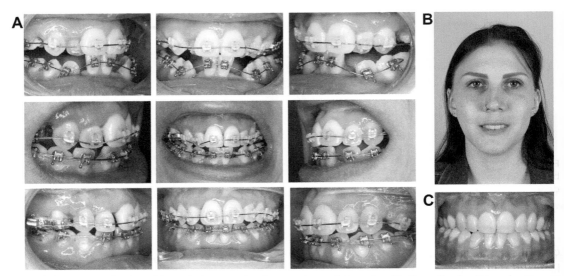

Fig. 8. (A) Postoperative instable occlusion requires frequent appointments with the orthodontist and active orthodontic treatment within a period of 6 months (listed chronologically from A to C), taking advantage of the RAP. (B). Clinical photo after a total treatment time of 12 months. (C). Final occlusion after a total treatment time of 12 months.

to achieve a stable postoperative occlusion without an increased risk of relapse. Patients presenting with severe crowding, buccally or palatally displaced canines, transversally collapsed dental arches, as well as exaggerated Curves of Spee in the maxilla and the mandible as seen in open bite deformities are the known challenges to go for a Surgery First approach. Classically, a palatally inclined dental arch in the premolar and molar areas of the maxilla with proclined upper incisors makes it difficult to set up a stable occlusion in surgical treatment planning,[28] and these dental obstacles were the logical consequence to promote Orthodontics First approach in the last century. However, we know that it is of major importance to correct the skeletal overgrowth in its original dimension[29] without any preoperative orthodontic camouflage to overcome muscle imbalances and achieve long-lasting stability. This is where the Surgery Early approach finds its place. In a digital dental setup in digital orthodontic software for fixed prebent appliances, the orthodontists create a piggyback occlusion with plausible dental arches which make it possible to put together a stable occlusion and have profound information about the final desired occlusion. The creation of a virtual occlusion in this preoperative 3D planning step has reached high predictability and accuracy. The only clinical limiting factor, especially in Caucasians in contrast to Asians,[6,30] is often the transverse width and the radius of the anterior segment,

as well as the inter-canine distance which are the obstacles in creating a proper overjet and overbite. A Surgery Early approach can be implemented for this condition. To manage these deficiencies, a premolar is extracted on each side,[31] and to start teeth alignment of the anterior segment from canine to canine, with the expansion of the radius of the anterior dental arch (**Fig. 10**). This is a short preoperative orthodontic treatment (up to 4 months), followed by early orthognathic surgery. An anatomically stable and rounded dental arch can be achieved surgically by segmentation of the maxilla via the extraction sockets (**Fig. 11A**). The segmental osteotomy allows 3D movements for harmonization of the occlusion (**Fig. 11**). The osteotomy sites may be grafted by autogenous bone harvested during the surgery, with 3 months of postoperative retention before orthodontic restarted. The described Surgery Early treatment protocol is particularly useful in open bite deformities with posterior overgrowth of the maxilla and collapsed dental arches with crowding. For the treatment planning, the surgeon first needs to define the final position and angulation of the upper front teeth, taking esthetics into consideration. The second decision is whether segmentation is required for the management of the transversal width. In case of upper arch segmentation without extractions is planned, presurgical orthodontics can create the space for the osteotomies by diverging the roots to reduce the risk of root

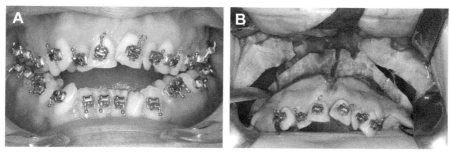

Fig. 9. (*A*) Open bite with transversal deficiency treated in Surgery First approach. The brackets were bonded before the surgery. (*B*). Segmented Le Fort I osteotomy in five pieces with additional midline osteotomy to avoid dental interferences at the canine area.

damage during the procedure. A short period of presurgical orthodontics may also help to reduce the need for midline segmentation of the anterior. A set of new prebent arch wires may be inserted intraoperatively or immediately postoperatively. The use of the robotically prebent arch wires is designed from the final aimed occlusion to the intra- or postoperative situation by backward-engineered digital planning and can help to control the outcome in cases of Surgery Early approach in an efficient and predictable manner.

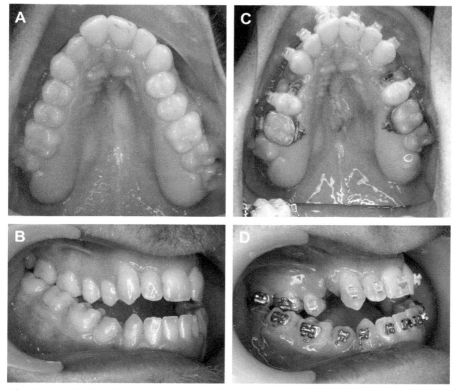

Fig. 10. (*A, B*) Patient with long-face syndrome, open bite, and narrowed dental arches. (*C, D*) Premolar extractions and starting of dental alignment to expand the inter-canine distance in a Surgery Early approach.

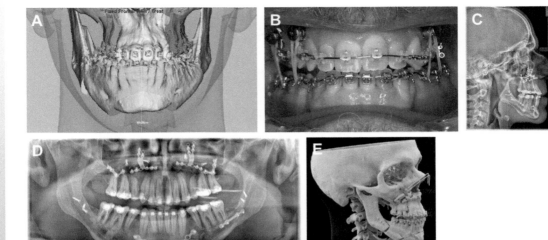

Fig. 11. (*A*) 3D virtual treatment plan with segmented LeFort I osteotomy, BSSO, and reduction genioplasty. (*B*). Occlusion postoperative 6 months showing the use of anchor screws. (*C*). Postoperative lateral cephalogram. (*D*). Postoperative orthopantomogram. (*E*). Postoperative 3D rendering of the CBCT.

SUMMARY

Surgery First approach should be in every orthognathic surgeon's portfolio by now. It should be in the best interest and well-being of our patients to keep the overall treatment times short, which include the orthodontic and surgical treatment periods. As elaborated extensively, this is only possible in a team approach between the surgeon and the orthodontist. In cases of primarily skeletal discrepancies in the relationship of the maxilla to the mandible with well-aligned dental arches, this is not challenging for postsurgical orthodontic treatment, and a stable postoperative occlusion is achievable. Alongside a planned occlusion, good function, and a patent airway, the surgical treatment plan is primarily oriented to improve esthetics by harmonizing the face and showing of teeth, with good lip projection, smile arch, and profile.[32] In patients with severe crowding, collapsed dental arches, exaggerated Curves of Spee and Wilson, and compensated angulations of the front teeth, careful planning is required to achieve a stable intraoperative and postoperative occlusion as well as the prediction of the final desired position of the teeth. Further, 3D virtual planning has improved surgical accuracy, yet the surgeons should also expect to learn from their experience of Surgery First or Surgery Early approaches, in particular the soft tissue changes and outcome. The creation of a digital dental setup, a 3D virtual simulation of a possible occlusion, and the production of postoperative robotic archwires from the final expected alignment through backward engineering have allowed a more predictable outcome in highly demanding cases.[33] To conclude, it is essential to have a thorough discussion between the surgeon, the orthodontist, and the patient to decide if a Surgery First approach, a Surgery Early approach, or the traditional Orthodontic First approach is most suitable for any orthognathic case in the treatment planning process.

CLINICS CARE POINTS

- The advantage of Surgery First or Early is a considerable reduction in overall treatment time due to the rapid acceleratory phenomenon and avoiding unfavorable resistance of musculature during the orthodontic treatment.

- When you come up with a treatment plan in a surgical orthognathic case, the Surgery First or Early approach should always be in the back of your head.

- The approach to make this decision should depend on the degree of deformity, crowding of the dental arches, exaggerated Curves of Spee, and whether the patient is reliable or not, to come in for his/her appointments. There must be a close relationship of trust between the surgeon and the orthodontist, who must be willing and capable to finish the case.

- The decision also depends on the manual skills and experience of the surgeon, because surgery compensates for prolonged orthodontic treatment by multiple segmentations of the maxilla for example.
- The promising development for the future is from Surgery First to Surgery Early taking advantage of digital preoperative planning and postoperative orthodontic finishing using robotically prebent archwires.

ADDITIONAL INFORMATION

All authors declare no potential conflicts of interest relevant to this. G.A. Millesi, M. Zimmermann, and M. Eltz contributed equally to the conceptualization, writing, and editing of the article.

All patients provided written informed consent for the publication and use of their images.

REFERENCES

1. Bell WH, Creekmore TD. Surgical-orthodontic correction of mandibular prognathism. Am J Orthod 1973;63(3):256–70.
2. Worms FW, Isaacson RJ, Speidel TM. Surgical orthodontic treatment planning: profile analysis and mandibular surgery. Angle Orthod 1976;46(1):1–25.
3. Oh COSH. Functional orthognathic surgery (1). Korean J Clin Orthod 2002;1:32–9.
4. Nagasaka H, Sugawara J, Kawamura H, et al. Surgery first" skeletal Class III correction using the Skeletal Anchorage System. J Clin Orthod 2009;43(2):97–105.
5. Sugawara J, Aymach Z, Nagasaka DH, et al. Surgery first" orthognathics to correct a skeletal class II malocclusion with an impinging bite. J Clin Orthod 2010;44(7):429–38.
6. Wang YC, Ko EW, Huang CS, et al. Comparison of transverse dimensional changes in surgical skeletal Class III patients with and without presurgical orthodontics. J Oral Maxillofac Surg 2010;68(8):1807–12.
7. Liao YF, Chiu YT, Huang CS, et al. Presurgical orthodontics versus no presurgical orthodontics: treatment outcome of surgical-orthodontic correction for skeletal class III open bite. Plast Reconstr Surg 2010;126(6):2074–83.
8. Luther F, Morris DO, Hart C. Orthodontic preparation for orthognathic surgery: how long does it take and why? A retrospective study. Br J Oral Maxillofac Surg 2003;41(6):401–6.
9. Proffit WR, Miguel JA. The duration and sequencing of surgical-orthodontic treatment. Int J Adult Orthodon Orthognath Surg 1995;10(1):35–42.
10. Hernández-Alfaro F, Guijarro-Martínez R, Molina-Coral A, et al. Surgery first" in bimaxillary orthognathic surgery. J Oral Maxillofac Surg 2011;69(6):e201–7.
11. Uribe F, Agarwal S, Shafer D, et al. Increasing orthodontic and orthognathic surgery treatment efficiency with a modified surgery-first approach. Am J Orthod Dentofacial Orthop 2015;148(5):838–48.
12. Baik HS, Han HK, Kim DJ, et al. Cephalometric characteristics of Korean Class III surgical patients and their relationship to plans for surgical treatment. Int J Adult Orthodon Orthognath Surg 2000;15(2):119–28.
13. Huang CS, Hsu SS, Chen YR. Systematic review of the surgery-first approach in orthognathic surgery. Biomed J 2014;37(4):184–90.
14. Huang X, Cen X, Sun W, et al. The impact of surgery-first approach on the oral health-related quality of life: a systematic review and meta-analysis. BMC Oral Health 2019;19(1):136.
15. Kole H. Surgical operations on the alveolar ridge to correct occlusal abnormalities. Oral Surg Oral Med Oral Pathol 1959;12(5):515–29. concl.
16. Wilcko WM, Wilcko T, Bouquot JE, et al. Rapid orthodontics with alveolar reshaping: two case reports of decrowding. Int J Periodontics Restorative Dent 2001;21(1):9–19.
17. Frost HM. The regional acceleratory phenomenon: a review. Henry Ford Hosp Med J 1983;31(1):3–9.
18. Yuan H, Zhu X, Lu J, et al. Accelerated orthodontic tooth movement following le fort I osteotomy in a rodent model. J Oral Maxillofac Surg 2014;72(4):764–72.
19. Liou EJ, Chen PH, Wang YC, et al. Surgery-first accelerated orthognathic surgery: postoperative rapid orthodontic tooth movement. J Oral Maxillofac Surg 2011;69(3):781–5.
20. Hernández-Alfaro F, Guijarro-Martínez R. On a definition of the appropriate timing for surgical intervention in orthognathic surgery. Int J Oral Maxillofac Surg 2014;43(7):846–55.
21. Sharma VK, Yadav K, Tandon P. An overview of surgery-first approach: Recent advances in orthognathic surgery. J Orthod Sci 2015;4(1):9–12.
22. Falter B, Schepers S, Vrielinck L, et al. Predicted versus executed surgical orthognathic treatment. J Craniomaxillofac Surg 2013;41(7):547–51.
23. Pelo S, Saponaro G, Patini R, et al. Risks in surgery-first orthognathic approach: complications of segmental osteotomies of the jaws. A systematic review. Eur Rev Med Pharmacol Sci 2017;21(1):4–12.
24. Hernández-Alfaro F, Guijarro-Martínez R, Peiró-Guijarro MA. Surgery first in orthognathic surgery: what have we learned? A comprehensive workflow based on 45 consecutive cases. J Oral Maxillofac Surg 2014;72(2):376–90.
25. Epker BN, Fish L. Surgical-orthodontic correction of open-bite deformity. Am J Orthod 1977;71(3):278–99.

26. Jong Woo Choi JYL. The surgery-first orthognathic approach. Singapore: Springer; 2021.

27. Turvey TA, Journot V, Epker BN. Correction of anterior open bite deformity: a study of tongue function, speech changes, and stability. J Maxillofac Surg 1976;4(2):93–101.

28. Yu HB, Mao LX, Wang XD, et al. The surgery-first approach in orthognathic surgery: a retrospective study of 50 cases. Int J Oral Maxillofac Surg 2015; 44(12):1463–7.

29. Behrman SJ, Behrman DA. Oral surgeons' considerations in surgical orthodontic treatment. Dent Clin North Am 1988;32(3):481–507.

30. Choi DS, Garagiola U, Kim SG. Current status of the surgery-first approach (part I): concepts and orthodontic protocols. Maxillofac Plast Reconstr Surg 2019;41(1):10.

31. Lee SJ, Kim TW, Nahm DS. Transverse implications of maxillary premolar extraction in Class III presurgical orthodontic treatment. Am J Orthod Dentofacial Orthop 2006;129(6):740–8.

32. Uribe FA, Farrell B. Surgery-first approach in the orthognathic patient. Oral Maxillofacial Surg Clin N Am 2020;32(1):89–103.

33. Baan F, van Meggelen EM, Verhulst AC, et al. Virtual occlusion in orthognathic surgery. Int J Oral Maxillofac Surg 2021;50(9):1219–25.

Zygoma and Mandibular Angle Reduction

Contouring Surgery to Correct the Square Face in Asians

Michael D. Han, DDS[a], Tae-Geon Kwon, DDS, PhD[b],*

KEYWORDS

- Malarplasty • Mandibular • Angle reduction • Zygoma • Contouring • Square face

KEY POINTS

- An oval facial contour is considered attractive in East Asia, and malar and gonial angle reduction is commonly sought by patients to achieve the oval facial look.
- Meticulous planning is critical in contouring surgeries to correct the square face. Preventing injury to adjacent structures and having a clear understanding of the postsurgical complications are essential.
- Potential complications of zygoma reduction include temporary sensory disturbance, cheek drooping, temporomandibular discomfort, and overcorrection or undercorrection.
- The position of the inferior alveolar nerve should be precisely noted in mandibular angle reduction. A palpable "secondary angle" or palpable masseter muscle attachments are potential concerns for patients.
- Application of three-dimensional surgical guides can enhance the accuracy of osteotomy line positioning and procedural safety.

INTRODUCTION

The facial shape of East Asians can be classified as round, square, or oval. Facial shape can influence an individual's preferred fashion style, such as hairstyle and type of glasses. Among the facial forms, the oval type is regarded as more favorable for women than the square type.[1] A prominent zygoma or angle is often associated with an intense or fierce image in East Asian countries. Similarly, a square face is regarded as more masculine than an oval one.[2] In East Asian countries including Korea and China, women prefer oval and slender faces ("V-shape"), as these facial types are considered more feminine. On the contrary, dolichocephalic craniofacial patterns are common in Western countries, as are deficient zygomas. As such, malar augmentation is more popular than malar reduction in Western countries, whereas in East Asian countries, reduction malarplasty, gonial angle reduction, genioplasty, chin, or body contouring surgery are frequently performed, either as independent procedures or as adjuncts during orthognathic surgery to achieve an oval facial contour. These procedures target the different parts of the face that contribute to a square look; prominence of the mandibular angle is influenced by the gonial angle and intergonial width, and a strong mandibular angle and the masseter muscles attenuate the malar prominence and give the face a squarer shape.

The current report focuses on the two most popular osseous contouring surgeries—reduction

a Department of Oral and Maxillofacial Surgery, College of Dentistry, University of Illinois Chicago, Chicago, IL 60612-7211, USA; b Department of Oral and Maxillofacial Surgery, School of Dentistry, Kyungpook National University, 2177 Dalgubeol-daero, Jung-gu, Daegu 41940, Republic of Korea
* Corresponding author.
E-mail address: kwondk@knu.ac.kr

Oral Maxillofacial Surg Clin N Am 35 (2023) 83–96
https://doi.org/10.1016/j.coms.2022.06.003
1042-3699/23/© 2022 Elsevier Inc. All rights reserved.

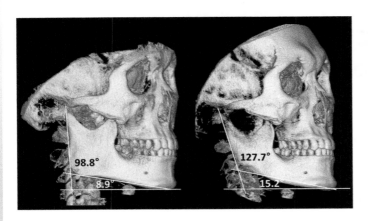

Fig. 1. The mandibular plane and the gonial angle are important references on the lateral view. The gonial angle (98.8°) and mandibular plane angle (8.9°) before surgery (*A*) were changed to 12.7° and 15.2°, respectively, after angle reduction (*B*).

malarplasty and mandibular angle reduction. Many techniques have been developed, and different osteotomy designs have been proposed to enhance outcomes and to minimize potential complications. Meticulous planning is especially important in osseous recontouring procedures to correct the square face type. Preventing injury to adjacent structures and having a clear understanding of the postsurgical complications are paramount. The purpose of this article is to review the surgical techniques and their considerations.

PREOPERATIVE EVALUATION AND PLANNING

Many patients can have soft tissue hypertrophy or atrophy, which together with the underlying osseous contours can influence their facial form. Evaluation of the square face should include a comprehensive examination of the midface, including the zygoma, masseter muscle, mandibular angle, and the vertical/horizontal position of the chin. Major features commonly seen in square-faced patients are (1) wide bilateral gonial width, (2) low gonial angle, (3) flat mandibular plane angle, (4) retrognathic appearance of the chin, and (5) short anterior face.[1] In the context of mandibular form, the square face is usually described as a low gonial angle deformity, with the gonial angle smaller than 110°[3] or 120°,[4] and the mandibular plane angle was smaller than 20°[3] or 30°[4] (**Fig. 1**).

When considering malarplasty, identifying key anatomic landmarks on photographs and three-dimensional computed tomography (3D-CT) is important. Cephalometric landmarks for evaluation of the zygoma are limited, and cephalometric norms have not yet been established. As such, subjective opinions or impressions from patient interviews are also important to complement the surgeon's impressions and clinical judgment. A key landmark when assessing malar form is the most prominent malar point (MP) on the soft

tissue, which usually lies in the posterior-superior quadrant of the intersection of two lines, called Hinderer's lines: (1) the line from the lateral canthus (Lc) to the lateral commissure and (2) the line from the superior aspect of the tragus to the alar base of nose.[5] According to Wilkinson, MP is located just distal to the Lc on a point one-third distance from Lc to the mandibular inferior border.[6] The facial width between the Lc, MP on both sides, and the most lateral point of the malar area (Zy) on both sides on the frontal view should be assessed. It should be noted that the MP and Zy do not always coincide (**Fig. 2**).

Reduction malarplasty directly influences the position of the MP, so appropriate positioning of the MP must be determined before surgery to determine the degree of zygomatic bone repositioning and volume reduction. When the MP is repositioned, the point is mobilized medially or posteriorly.[7] Occasionally, patients with normal malar projections can appear to have relatively prominent projections because of depressions in the frontal or cheek regions. In such cases, soft tissue contouring of these areas must be performed instead of malar reduction.[8] In addition to changing the position of the MP, malarplasty can change the lateral prominence of the zygomatic arch. When the zygomatic arch is prominent, it can be rotated inward to decrease the lateral projection.

When planning mandibular recontouring, angle reduction is efficient for correcting mild to moderately prominent mandibular angles. However, in patients with a wide intergonial width, a low gonial angle and a flat mandibular plane at the same time, a long-curved osteotomy and a mandibular outer cortex splitting osteotomy are required. In patients with retrognathic or prognathic chins, the correction of skeletal problems using orthognathic surgery or genioplasty is necessary in combination with angle reduction.[9,10]

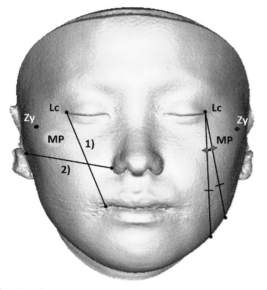

Fig. 2. The most prominent malar point in the soft tissue (MP) usually lies in the posterio-superior quadrant (yellow circle) of the intersection of Hinderer's lines: 1) line from the lateral canthus (Lc) to the lateral commissure and (2) line from the superior aspect of the tragus to the alar base of nose. MP (red dot) also lies just distal to the Lc on a point one-third distance from Lc to mandibular inferior border. MP does not always same to the most lateral point of malar area (Zy, blue dot).

Because of the multifactorial nature of the etiology of the square face, for some patients, multiple surgical techniques are required to correct these problems. Because of the irreversible nature of reductive facial recontouring procedures, thorough patient communication is paramount.

REDUCTION MALARPLASTY
Surgical Technique

As Onizuka and colleagues[11] first reported bony shaving of the malar body via an intraoral approach, numerous surgeons have reported a variety of techniques for reduction malarplasty. The design of the osteotomy is largely divided into zygoma shaving,[12] I-shaped osteotomy,[12–18] L-shaped osteotomy,[12,16,19–31] and their modifications.[12,16,17,32–34] Shaving the outer cortex of the zygoma with a bur (without zygoma osteotomy) cannot decrease the bizygomatic distance. In addition, it is difficult to maintain malar symmetry or a natural malar contours with this technique. Therefore, the clinical use of zygoma shaving is limited.[35]

The intraoral approach is now the standard procedure to expose the anterior zygomatic body. To perform the osteotomy at the posterior zygomatic arch, coronal,[16] preauricular,[12,13,20,23,27] sideburn,[14,17,22,24–26,28,33,36] temporal,[37] and intraoral-only approaches have been used (with[38–40] or without[15,16,19,21,30,32,34,41] endoscopy). Currently, the intraoral with or without sideburn approaches are gaining popularity. In these procedures, the osteotomized zygoma is repositioned without fixation[13,15,16,18,23] or with anterior/posterior fixation.[12,14,16,17,19–22,24,26–28,30,32–34,36] The most popular fixation is miniplate fixation at the zygomatico-maxillary osteotomy site. The approaches can be determined by the surgeon's preference and surgical experience. The types of osteotomies and the approaches used are summarized in **Table 1**.

Recent studies have more frequently used the L-shaped malarplasty than the I-shaped osteotomy. The major advantage of L-shaped osteotomy

Table 1
Type of osteotomy, approach, and osseous fixation for reduction malarplasty

Design of Osteotomy Line	Approach	Fixation Method

• I-shaped osteotomy[1–7]
• Modified I-shaped osteotomy[5,6]
• L-shaped osteotomy[1,5,8–20]
• Modified L-shaped osteotomy[1,21–23]
	• Coronal[5]
	• Preauricular only[2]
	• Intraoral/preauricular[1,9,12,16]
	• Intraoral/sideburn[3,6,11,13–15,17,22,24]
	• Intraoral/temporal[25]
	• Intraoral only[4,5,8,10,19,21,23,26]
	• Intraoral (endoscopy)[27–29]
		• Greenstick fracture[26,30,31]
		• No fixation[2,4,5,7,12]
		• Osteotomy and fixation
		  1 point (ant or post)[a]
		    fixation[1,3,6,8–10,13,17,19,21–23]
		  2 point (ant and post)[a]
		    fixation[5,11,15,16,24]

Ant, zygomatico-maxillary buttress; post, posterior aspect of zygomatic arch.

is that the location of the osteotomy lies in the anterior region of the zygomaxillary suture region and is easy to access during fixation of the osteotomized segments. Another advantage of L-shaped osteotomy is that the most prominent aspect of the zygoma is included in the site of bone reduction in L-shaped osteotomy. A comparison of the two techniques is presented in **Fig. 3** and **Table 2**.

Surgical Steps for L-Shaped Osteotomy

Reduction malarplasty is a blind approach with limited visualization. The surgical steps of L-shaped osteotomy for malar reduction are as follows:

1. 3D planning and simulation:
   Using cone beam computed tomography (CBCT) data, 3D surgical planning is performed to simulate the amount of bone volume reduction and the direction and magnitude of the mobilized segment (**Fig. 4**).

2. Mucogingival incision:
   An incision is made on the buccal sulcus from the canine to the molar.

3. Subperiosteal reflection:
   Mucoperiosteal reflection is carried out to the infraorbital foramen, zygomatic body, maxilla anterior wall, posterior to anterior part of the zygomatic arch, and superiorly to the junction of the lateral orbital rim and the zygomatic arch.

4. Oblique osteotomy:
   a. Two oblique osteotomies start from the junction of the lateral orbital rim and the zygomatic arch.
   b. The line extends anterio-medially to a point 5 mm inferior to the infraorbital foramen. The distance between the two oblique osteotomy lines does not need to be large.[28] The main purpose of this ostectomy is to facilitate the medialization of the zygoma body, rather than to allow volumetric reduction.[6]

5. Vertical osteotomy:

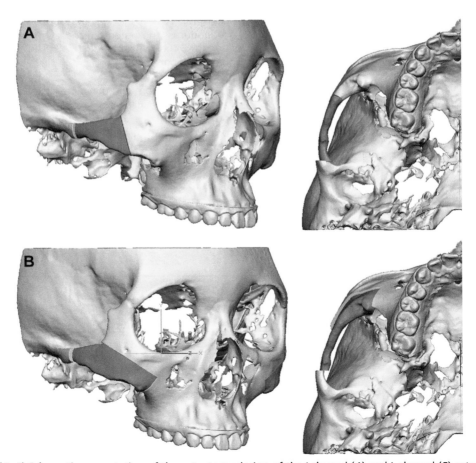

Fig. 3. (*A*, *B*) Schematic presentation of the osteotomy design of the I-shaped (*A*) and L-shaped (*B*) osteotomies.

Table 2
Comparison of I-shaped versus L-shaped osteotomy

	I-Shaped Osteotomy[1,2]	L-Shaped Osteotomy[1,19]
Outline of osteotomy	Anterior cut: vertical I-shaped cut Posterior cut: zygomatic arch cut Mobilize and displace the zygoma antero-medially; interosseous fixation	Anterior cut: oblique (long) + vertical (short) Posterior cut: zygomatic arch cut Mobilize and displace the zygoma antero-medially; interosseous fixation
Indications	Wide zygomatic arch and lateral protrusion of the zygomatic body (when the zygomatic body is not prominent)	Protrusion of the zygomatic body and arch (serious protrusion of the anterior part of the arch exists)
Effects	Narrowing of the wide zygomatic arches Reduce the anterior protrusion of the zygomatic body	Large amount of bone removal Significant medial reduction can be achieved
Precautions	Possible bulging of the most prominent part of the zygomatic arch even after surgery	More infraorbital reflection Possibility of inferior displacement (needs rigid internal fixation)

The vertical osteotomy line (the short limb of the L-osteotomy) is located near the zygomaticomaxillary suture, nearly at a right angle to the oblique osteotomy line. The osteotomized segment of zygomatic bone is then removed.

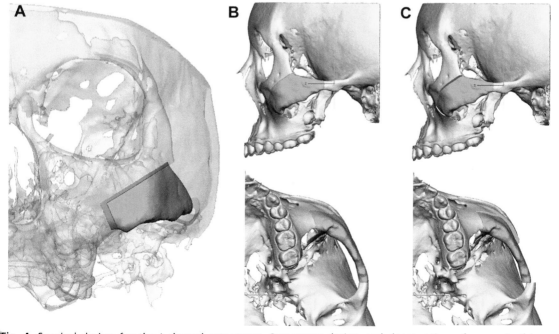

Fig. 4. Surgical design for the L-shaped osteotomy. Osteotomy design and demarcation of amount of bone removal (*A*), before (*B*), and after (*C*) the reduction malarplasty from the lateral (upper), and submentovertical views (lower).

6. Zygomatic arch osteotomy:
   A preauricular sideburn incision, 1 cm in length, is made 20 mm anterior to the tragus. The periosteum above the zygomatic arch is reached using blunt dissection. Zygomatic arch osteotomy is performed anterior to the anterior border of the articular tubercle.
   The periosteum of the inner and outer sides of the osteotomy site is reflected, and the reciprocating saw is used from the inner side to the outer side to prevent damage to the neurovascular structures.
7. Mobilization and fixation:
   After confirming the mobilization of the osteotomized zygoma, the segment is fixated in the planned position with a plate and screws, anteriorly with a miniplate, posteriorly with a microplate, or without fixation.
8. Smoothening of bony step:
   The residual bony step is smoothened with a bur.

Complications in Reduction Malarplasty and Their Managements

Although malarplasty is a safe procedure when performed by experienced surgeons, it carries the risk of many complications compared with other surgical procedures. One major postoperative complication is zygomatic nonunion.[42] To correct this, a coronal approach is required to access the nonunion site to remove fibrotic scar tissue and to achieve bony contact after mobilization of the segment. If there is a large bony gap, bone grafting should be considered.

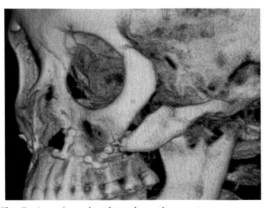

Fig. 5. A patient developed continuous temporomandibular joint pain on the left side after previous malarplasty. Postoperative CT showing zygomatic bone displacement and nonunion at 1 year after the surgery.

Table 3
Complications and management

Complications	Management
Malunion or nonunion	Secondary surgery and refixation
Mouth-opening restriction/ Temporomandibular joint pain	Physiotherapy, medication, evaluation of the status of bony union
Cheek drooping	Secondary surgery or face lifting
Transient intraoprbital hypoesthesia	None, or medication
Transient facial nerve injury	None, or medication
Asymmetry, overcorrection or undercorrection	None, or secondary surgery, if needed

Postoperative trismus or temporomandibular joint problems commonly occur after surgery. This is mainly attributed to malunion of the zygoma, displacement of the zygomatic arch, rotation of the zygoma, or floating zygoma from fixation failure. These malunions are also accompanied by cheek ptosis and/or malar depression. Repositioning of the displaced zygomatic complex must be performed via a coronal approach.[43] For trismus after surgery, active mouth-opening exercises are recommended after 2 to 3 weeks following surgery.

Cheek drooping or sagging can be seen when there is inferior displacement and external rotation of the mobilized zygomatic complex (**Fig. 5**). As the traction force of the masseter muscle is strong, osseous fixation must be sufficiently strong to resist the masseter muscle force during mastication.[43,44] It has been suggested that high-level fixation on the superior region of the zygomatic bone is favorable to low-level fixation near the zygomatico-maxillary buttress to prevent malunion or nonunion caused by strong masseter muscle action.[29] Other complications include undercorrection or overcorrection and postsurgical asymmetry, which can be corrected by reoperation or a separate secondary corrective procedure.[45] Complications and management after malarplasty are summarized in **Table 3**.

ANGLE REDUCTION
Surgical Technique

A prominent mandibular angle is not considered attractive in Asian women. Various surgical techniques have been introduced to achieve oval and slender mandibular angles and correct square-shaped faces. The aim of angle reduction is to achieve a natural, balanced, and symmetric mandibular outline in both the frontal and lateral views while minimizing surgical complications. Various surgical techniques have been proposed to improve the prominent angles in terms of width control from frontal view and increase the gonial angle from the lateral view. Classical angle reduction is still popular in many practices, and its modifications are increasingly being applied.[46–49] The indications and anticipated effects of different surgical techniques are compared in **Table 4**. A schematic of angle reduction and its modifications is shown in **Fig. 6**.

Surgical Procedure of Angle Reduction with 3D-Printed Surgical Guide

In this section, angle reduction using a 3D-printed surgical guide fabricated by computer-aided design and manufacturing (CAD/CAM) is demonstrated. As the mandibular cortex is thick and hard, it takes time to penetrate bicortically with an oscillating saw blade. Making cortical holes along the planned osteotomy line before osteotomy is helpful while handling the saw. Subsequently, the oscillating saw can follow the small marking holes[50,51] However, if a 3D-printed surgical guide is used, marking holes are not required, and the operation time is reduced. Because it is easy to follow the surgical guide during osteotomy, the surgical steps are more safely executed. The surgical steps for angle reduction with a 3D-printed surgical guide are summarized as follows:

1. Fabrication of 3D surgical guide:
   a. 3D surgical guides are designed with a virtual surgery software using the patient's CBCT data.
   b. The outline of the virtual guides is established after confirmation of the position of the inferior alveolar nerve and the virtual osteotomy line (**Fig. 7**).
   c. The guides are designed based on surgeon preference (**Figs. 8 and 9**). In this example, two types of the CAD/CAM-fabricated surgical splint are made—"superior-based" and "inferior-based" angle reduction guides (FACEGIDE, MegaGen implant, Daegu, South Korea). The 3D guides were designed to slightly wrap around the posterior and inferior margins of the mandibular angle and with holes for temporary screw fixation.
   d. After fabrication, the surgical guides are inspected for possible discrepancies with the 3D design.

2. Mucogingival incision:
   An incision is made on the buccal sulcus inferior to the mucogingival junction from the mandibular first premolar to the external oblique ridge.
3. Subperiosteal reflection:
   a. Confirm the location of the mental nerve, without reflecting all the periosteum around it.
   b. Visualize the ascending ramus, mandibular body, and gonial angle. Completely detach the masseteric insertion at the gonial angle.
   c. Exercise special caution to avoid injury to the following major neurovascular structures during the flap reflection and osteotomy: (1) ascending ramus—retromandibular vein, (2) mandibular body—mental nerve, and (3) antegonial notch—facial nerve, facial vein.
4. Adaptation of the 3D surgical guide to surgical field:
   The 3D-printed surgical guide is placed to ensure excellent adaptation on all indexed surfaces. The "inferior-based" angle reduction guide is adapted to the outer side of mandibular angle. Subsequently, correct position and stability of the surgical guide are confirmed. Right-angled instrumentation is used to fixate the surgical guide to the mandibular angle (**Fig. 10A**).
5. Angle ostectomy:
   Angle ostectomy is performed with an oscillating saw along the upper margin of the surgical guide (**Fig. 10B**). After the mandibular angle is completely cut, the osteotomized mandibular angle with the surgical guide and screw is removed (**Fig. 10C**).
6. Smoothening of bony step:
   The existing secondary angle or bony prominence is smoothened with a bur. The mandibular lateral cortex is reduced to the planned extent. The mental nerve is carefully protected during surgery.

Complications in Mandibular Angle Reduction and Their Management

Table 5 provides a list of complications and representative managements after angle reduction. Even though most patients are satisfied with the results of angle reduction, as with other contouring surgeries, this procedure is not free of complications. Various rates of complications after angle reduction have been reported in the literature, ranging from 5.9% to 9.9%.[52–54] The most commonly reported complication in these reports was numbness, which ranged from 0.8% to 4.9%[52–54] of all patients who received angle

Table 4
Angle reduction and its modifications

	Angle Reduction[32]	Curved Ostectomy[33,34]	"V-Line" Ostectomy[34,35]	Lateral Cortex Ostectomy[34,36]
Outline of osteotomy	Curvilinear ostectomy between the two points; point 1 = intersection of line extending from occlusal plane and posterior ramal border. Point 2 = intersection of perpendicular line along the anterior ramal border and inferior mandibular border.	Extended curvilinear angle reduction; point 1 extending more superiorly and point 2 more anteriorly to the inferior border just behind the mental foramen.	Straight line resection of the inferior border from the menton to the posterior edge of the ascending ramus (with reciprocating saw)	Horizontal cut made at least 10 mm inferior to the sigmoid notch; anterior vertical cut made 10 mm posterior to the mental foramen.
Indications	1. Low gonial angle 2. Mild or moderately increased mandibular width	1. Low gonial angle 2. Moderately increased mandibular width	1. Low gonial angle 2. Small mandibular plane angle and normal mandibular width	1. Normal gonial angle 2. Increased mandibular width
	A combination of surgical techniques can be applied to a patient according to the individual characteristics of the prominent mandibular angle. Combined genioplasty can be performed with angle reduction.			
Effects	Increases gonial angle and reduces the prominent bulging of the mandibular angle, but does not dramatically improve the width		Increase steepness of the mandibular plane angle, increases gonial angle	Narrow the mandibular width by removing prominent bone affecting the mandibular width
Precautions	Retromandibular vein, facial artery injury, and IAN damage during osteotomy	Retromandibular vein, facial artery injury, and IAN damage during osteotomy	Possibility of IAN transection, especially at the mandibular body areas.	IAN damage during drilling and ostectomy.

Abbreviation: IAN, inferior alveolar nerve.

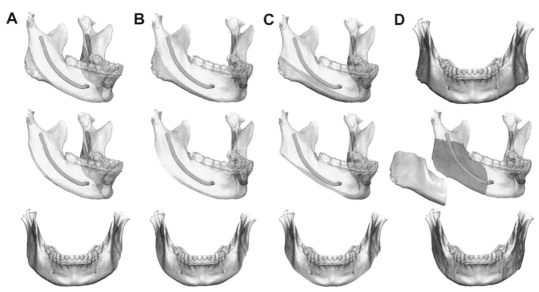

Fig. 6. Schematic of classical angle reduction (*A*), curved angle ostectomy (*B*), "V-line" ostectomy (*C*), and lateral cortex ostectomy (*D*).

reduction. There was better sensory recovery when neurotrauma resulted from traction or compression, as compared with when complete transection of the inferior alveolar nerve was observed. In the author's experience, surgeons need to be aware of a greater risk of inferior alveolar nerve transection when performing a straight-line V-line ostectomy. As the inferior alveolar nerve does not have a straight-line course, this straight-line ostectomy can directly injure the curved inferior alveolar nerve in the mandibular body (**Fig. 11**).

To avoid overcorrection or undercorrection or postoperative asymmetry in the gonial and secondary angles, all ostectomy lines should be clearly visualized after finishing the osteotomy. A "second mandibular angle" deformity can be encountered, especially when a straight line ostectomy is performed.[55] To solve this problem, multiple osteotomy[56] or lateral cortex osteotomy[55] have been proposed. Based on the author's experience, a reciprocating rasp and a round bur are helpful in smoothing the secondary angle. Palpation of the osteotomy edge can help in identifying a secondary angle before and after smoothening.

Using an intraoral approach poses several challenges because of fundamental limitations in

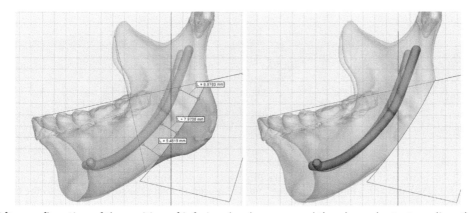

Fig. 7. After confirmation of the position of inferior alveolar nerve and the planned ostectomy line, the outline of the virtual guide was established (FACEGIDE, MegaGen implant, Daegu, South Korea).

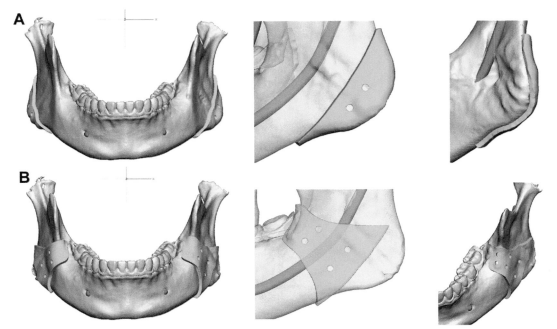

Fig. 8. (*A, B*) Two types of the CAD/CAM-fabricated surgical splint were made: "superior-based" (*A*) and "inferior-based" (*B*) angle reduction guides.

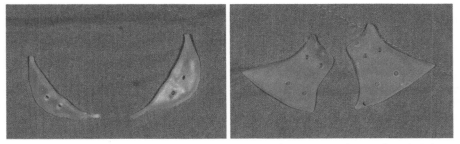

Fig. 9. Three-dimensional guides with holes for temporary screw fixation was designed to slightly wrap around the inferior or superior margin and of mandibular angle.

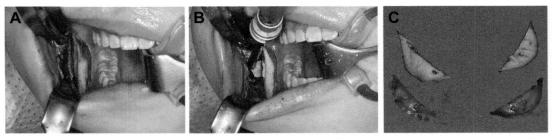

Fig. 10. (*A–C*) Adaptation of the 3D surgical guide. Right-angled drill and screw driver (Stryker Craniomaxillofacial, Portage, MI, USA) and one 5 mm screw on each sides was used to fixate the surgical guide to the mandibular angle (*left*). The angle ostectomy was performed with an oscillating saw along the upper margin of the surgical guide (*middle*). After the mandibular angle is completely cut, the osteotomized mandibular angle with the surgical guide and screw is removed (*right*).

Table 5
Complications and management

Complications	Management
Lower lip numbness	Prevention is the best measure
Severe swelling after surgery	Investigate any potential source of secondary bleeding, consider hematoma evacuation immediately after surgery
Massive bleeding	Compression, application of hemostatic agent, direct ligation, angiographic embolization, if needed
Infection	Antibiotics, inspect focus of infection, incision, and drainage
Mouth corner damage/scar	None, scar revision, if needed
Secondary angle formation	Secondary surgery, if needed
Subcondylar fracture	Open reduction internal fixation/closed treatment

visualization and access. Because osteotomies in the posterior ramus are done in a blind manner, special care should be taken to avoid injuring the retromandibular vein or the facial artery. Occasionally, continuous bone bleeding can occur, which can be controlled by the application of resorbable bone wax. When the ostectomy encompasses the posterior ramal surface and the inferior border of the mandible, the limited visualization and access as well as parallax make it challenging to control the direction of the oscillating saw. The osteotomy line at the posterior border of the ascending ramus is frequently misdirected vertically and can reach the sigmoid notch, resulting in a subcondylar fracture[1,57](**Fig. 12**). Also, sometimes the shank of the oscillating saw can contact the mouth corner, causing iatrogenic injury.

FUTURE CONSIDERATIONS IN MALARPLASTY AND ANGLE REDUCTION

Minimally invasive endoscopic surgery has been extensively applied for malarplasty[31,38–40] and angle reduction.[40] Using an endoscope, the surgeon can more actively visualize the narrow operative field. Reports show encouraging results, with successful osteotomies through conservative incisions leaving minimally visible scars when using endoscopic techniques.

Another new trend involves the application of computer-assisted surgical simulations. Recent advancements in computer-aided surgery have been actively applied to malarplasty and mandibular angle reduction. For malarplasty, a customized surgical guides based on 3D virtual surgery had been introduced.[58,59] Regarding mandibular

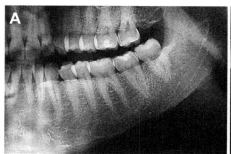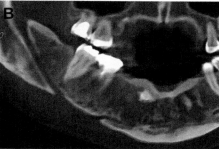

Fig. 11. (*A, B*) Imaging of two patients referred for neurosensory deficit following straight-line V-line ostectomies. Inferior alveolar nerve transection was noted in both patients (*right* and *left*). Straight-line osteotomy directly injured the curve-shaped inferior alveolar nerve at the mandibular body.

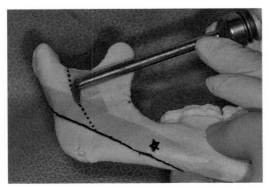

Fig. 12. Following the rotation arc of the oscillating saw can lead to a ramal or subcondylar fracture.

angle reduction, it has been reported that computer-assisted surgery and 3D-printed surgical guide can minimize the surgical discrepancy and increase safety.[60]

SUMMARY

Angle reduction and reduction malarplasty are the most popular bone contouring surgeries to correct square-shaped faces in East Asians. These procedures are not only performed in young women, with increasing demand in male and older adults as well. Before performing surgery, meticulous planning and a thorough understanding of surgical techniques, related anatomic structures, and potential risks are necessary to achieve a harmonious face while ensuring surgical safety.

CLINICS CARE POINTS

> The following guiding principles need to be emphasized for clinical care for malar and mandibular angle reduction:
>
> - No floating zygoma.
>
>   Osteotomized zygoma need to be rigidly fixated in the planned position with a plate and screws after reduction malarplasty. These can minimize potential cheek drooping related with masseteric traction subsequent inferior displacement of zygoma.
>
> - Aware of the width from the frontal view.
>
>   When performing mandibular angle reduction, not only the gonial angle from the lateral view but also the frontal intergonial width should be considered. Classical angle reduction, curved angle ostectomy, "V-line" ostectomy, and lateral cortex ostectomy can be used based on the patients' characteristics of mandibular angle prominence.

> - No damage to inferior alveolar nerve.
>
>   Inferior alveolar nerve transection should be avoided during extensive angle reduction, especially when performing straight-line "V-line" osteotomy.

DISCLOSURE

There are no commercial or financial conflicts of interest or any funding sources for all authors.

REFERENCES

1. Li X, Hsu Y, Hu J, et al. Comprehensive consideration and design for treatment of square face. J Oral Maxillofac Surg 2013;71(10):1761.e1-4.
2. Hage JJ, Becking AG, de Graaf FH, et al. Gender-confirming facial surgery: considerations on the masculinity and femininity of faces. Plast Reconstr Surg 1997;99(7):1799–807.
3. Li J, Hsu Y, Khadka A, et al. Surgical designs and techniques for mandibular contouring based on categorisation of square face with low gonial angle in orientals. J Plast Reconstr Aesthet Surg 2012; 65(1):e1–8.
4. Hsu YC, Li J, Hu J, et al. Correction of square jaw with low angles using mandibular "V-line" ostectomy combined with outer cortex ostectomy. Oral Surg Oral Med Oral Pathol Oral Radiol Endod 2010; 109(2):197–202.
5. Hinderer UT. Malar implants for improvement of the facial appearance. Plast Reconstr Surg 1975;56(2): 157–65.
6. Wilkinson TS. Complications in aesthetic malar augmentation. Plast Reconstr Surg 1983;71(5): 643–9.
7. Gao ZW, Wang WG, Zeng G, et al. A modified reduction malarplasty utilizing 2 oblique osteotomies for prominent zygomatic body and arch. J Craniofac Surg 2013;24(3):812–7.
8. Uhm KI, Lew JM. Prominent zygoma in Orientals: classification and treatment. Ann Plast Surg 1991; 26(2):164–70.
9. Kim SK, Han JJ, Kim JT. Classification and treatment of prominent mandibular angle. Aesthet Plast Surg 2001;25(5):382–7.
10. Shao Z, Peng Q, Xu Y, et al. Combined long-curved ostectomy in the inferior mandibular border and angle of the mandible with splitting corticectomy for reduction of the lower face. Aesthet Plast Surg 2011;35(3):382–9.
11. Onizuka T, Watanabe K, Takasu K, et al. Reduction malar plasty. Aesthet Plast Surg 1983;7(2):121–5.
12. Chen T, Hsu Y, Li J, et al. Correction of zygoma and zygomatic arch protrusion in East Asian individuals

Oral Surg Oral Med Oral Pathol Oral Radiol Endod 2011;112(3):307–14.

13. Rhee DY, Kim SH, Shin DH, et al. Lateral facial contouring via a single preauricular incision. J Plast Reconstr Aesthet Surg 2012;65(8):e205–12.

14. Shao Z, Xie Y, Yu B, et al. A new assisted fixation technique to prevent zygoma displacement in malar reduction. Aesthet Plast Surg 2013;37(4):692–6.

15. Shim BK, Shin HS, Nam SM, et al. Real-time navigation-assisted orthognathic surgery. J Craniofac Surg 2013;24(1):221–5.

16. Zhang Y, Tang M, Jin R, et al. Comparison of three techniques of reduction malarplasty in zygomaticus and massateric biomechanical changes and relevant complications. Ann Plast Surg 2014;73(2): 131–6.

17. Baek W, Woo T, Kim YS, et al. Reduction malarplasty by bidirectional wedge ostectomy or two percutaneous osteotomies according to zygoma protrusion type. J Craniomaxillofac Surg 2016;44(10):1662–9.

18. Li Q, Gao B, Li K, et al. A Novel Technique for Reduction Malarplasty by Inward Displacement of Infractured Zygomatic Arch Without Fixation. J Oral Maxillofac Surg 2017;75(12):2658–66.

19. Hong SE, Liu SY, Kim JT, et al. Intraoral zygoma reduction using L-shaped osteotomy. J Craniofac Surg 2014;25(3):758–61.

20. Ma YQ, Zhu SS, Li JH, et al. Reduction malarplasty using an L-shaped osteotomy through intraoral and sideburns incisions. Aesthet Plast Surg 2011;35(2): 237–41.

21. Tan W, Niu F, Yu B, et al. Feasibility of absorbable plates and screws for fixation in reduction malarplasty with L-shaped osteotomy. J Craniofac Surg 2011;22(2):546–50.

22. Choung JW. Rotation technique of reduction malar plasty. J Craniofac Surg 2015;26(1):238–9.

23. Lin LX, Yuan JL, Wang YT, et al. A New Infracture Technique for Reduction Malarplasty with an L-Shaped Osteotomy Line. Med Sci Monit 2015;21: 1949–54.

24. Zou C, Niu F, Liu JF, et al. Application of Computer Techniques in Correcting Mild Zygomatic Assymetry With Unilateral Reduction Malarplasty. J Craniofac Surg 2015;26(6):2002–4.

25. Lee TS. Standardization of surgical techniques used in facial bone contouring. J Plast Reconstr Aesthet Surg 2015;68(12):1694–700.

26. Hwang CH, Lee MC. Reduction malarplasty using a zygomatic arch-lifting technique. J Plast Reconstr Aesthet Surg 2016;69(6):809–18.

27. Kim TG, Cho YK. A New Double Trapezoid-Shaped Osteotomy for Reduction Malarplasty. J Craniofac Surg 2016;27(1):87–93.

28. Yang HW, Hong JJ, Koo YT. Reduction Malarplasty that Uses Malar Setback Without Resection of Malar Body Strip. Aesthet Plast Surg 2017;41(4):910–8.

29. Kim JW, Hwang W. Optimal Fixation Location in Intraoral Reduction Malarplasty Using an L-Shaped Osteotomy. J Craniofac Surg 2019;30(8):2490–2.

30. Kim YH, Seul JH. Reduction malarplasty through an intraoral incision: a new method. Plast Reconstr Surg 2000;106(7):1514–9.

31. Lee JS, Kim EH, Lee SH. Endoscopically assisted malarplasty: L-rotation technique. J Stomatol Oral Maxillofac Surg 2021;122(3):229–34.

32. Kook MS, Jung S, Park HJ, et al. Reduction malarplasty using modified L-shaped osteotomy. J Oral Maxillofac Surg 2012;70(1):e87–91.

33. Nakanishi Y, Nagasao T, Shimizu Y, et al. The boomerang osteotomy – a new method of reduction malarplasty. J Plast Reconstr Aesthet Surg 2012; 65(5):e111–20.

34. Zou C, Niu F, Liu J, et al. Midface contour change after reduction malarplasty with a modified L-shaped osteotomy: a surgical outcomes study. Aesthet Plast Surg 2014;38(1):177–83.

35. Kim YH, Cho BC, Lo LJ. Facial contouring surgery for asians. Semin Plast Surg 2009;23(1):22–31.

36. Lee SW, Myung Y, Jeong YW. Bone Resection Versus Setback in Reduction Malarplasty: A Quantitative Analysis of the Migration of the Summit of the Zygoma. Aesthet Plast Surg 2016;40(3):349–59.

37. Ma F, Tang S. Zygomatic arch reduction and malarplasty with multiple osteotomies: its geometric considerations. Aesthet Plast Surg 2014;38(6):1143–50.

38. Kim JW. Laser-assisted endoscopic reduction malarplasty in Asians: quick combined surgery. Aesthet Plast Surg 1998;22(4):289–97.

39. Lee JS, Kang S, Kim YW. Endoscopically assisted malarplasty: one incision and two dissection planes. Plast Reconstr Surg 2003;111(1):461–7 [discussion: 468].

40. Wu G, Zhou B, Chen X, et al. Endoscopic-Assisted Intraoral Three-Dimensional Reduction Mandibuloplasty. Ann Plast Surg 2015;75(1):10–8.

41. Lee JG, Park YW. Intraoral approach for reduction malarplasty: a simple method. Plast Reconstr Surg 2003;111(1):453–60.

42. Myung Y, Kwon H, Lee SW, et al. Postoperative Complications Associated With Reduction Malarplasty via Intraoral Approach: A Meta Analysis. Ann Plast Surg 2017;78(4):371–8.

43. Baek RM, Kim J, Kim BK. Three-dimensional assessment of zygomatic malunion using computed tomography in patients with cheek ptosis caused by reduction malarplasty. J Plast Reconstr Aesthet Surg 2012;65(4):448–55.

44. Lee YH, Lee SW. Zygomatic nonunion after reduction malarplasty. J Craniofac Surg 2009;20(3): 849–52.

45. Rodman R. Cosmetic bone contouring. Curr Opin Otolaryngol Head Neck Surg 2017;25(4):337–40.

46. Liu D, Huang J, Shan L, et al. Intraoral curved ostectomy for prominent mandibular angle by grinding, contiguous drilling, and chiseling. J Craniofac Surg 2011;22(6):2109–13.

47. Song G, Zong X, Guo X, et al. Single-Stage Mandibular Curved Ostectomy on Affected Side Combined with Bilateral Outer Cortex Grinding for Correction of Facial Asymmetry: Indications and Outcomes. Aesthet Plast Surg 2019;43(3):733–41.

48. Khadka A, Hsu Y, Hu J, et al. Clinical observations of correction of square jaw in East Asian individuals. Oral Surg Oral Med Oral Pathol Oral Radiol Endod 2011;111(4):428–34.

49. Han K, Kim J. Reduction mandibuloplasty: ostectomy of the lateral cortex around the mandibular angle. J Craniofac Surg 2001;12(4):314–25.

50. Gao B, He J, Xie F, et al. Stamp Perforation" Technique for Correction of Prominent Mandibular Angle: 10 Years of Experience in Mandibular Reshaping in Asians. Ann Plast Surg 2017;78(6):618–22.

51. Park JL, Oh CH, Hwang K, et al. Burring and holes connecting ostectomy for the correction of prominent mandible angle. J Craniofac Surg 2014;25(3): 1025–7.

52. Chen H, Sun J, Wang J. Reducing Prominent Mandibular Angle Osteotomy Complications: 10-Year Retrospective Review. Ann Plast Surg 2018; 81(6S Suppl 1):S5–9.

53. Yoon ES, Seo YS, Kang DH, et al. Analysis of incidences and types of complications in mandibular angle ostectomy in Koreans. Ann Plast Surg 2006; 57(5):541–4.

54. Kang M. Incidence of Complications Associated with Mandibuloplasty: A Review of 588 Cases over 5 Years. Plast Reconstr Surg Glob Open 2014;2(4): e139.

55. Gui L, Yu D, Zhang Z, et al. Intraoral one-stage curved osteotomy for the prominent mandibular angle: a clinical study of 407 cases. Aesthet Plast Surg 2005;29(6):552–7.

56. Baek SM, Baek RM, Shin MS. Refinement in aesthetic contouring of the prominent mandibular angle. Aesthet Plast Surg 1994;18(3):283–9.

57. Hwang K, Han JY, Kil MS, et al. Treatment of condyle fracture caused by mandibular angle ostectomy. J Craniofac Surg 2002;13(5):709–12.

58. Ha SH, Jung S, Choi JY. Reduction Malarplasty Using Customized Surgical Stent Based on 3D Virtual Surgery, CAD/CAM, and 3D Printing Technology: Case Series. J Craniofac Surg 2021. https://doi.org/10.1097/SCS.0000000000008430.

59. Kang SH, Tak HJ, Kim HJ, et al. Reduction malarplasty using a simulated surgical guide for asymmetric/prominent zygoma. Head Face Med 2022; 18(1):11.

60. Yi CR, Choi JW. Three-Dimension-Printed Surgical Guide for Accurate and Safe Mandibuloplasty in Patients With Prominent Mandibular Angles. J Craniofac Surg 2019;30(7):1979–81.

Genioplasty in Contemporary Orthognathic Surgery

Mrunalini Ramanathan, MDS, PhD Resident[a],
Elavenil Panneerselvam, MDS, MBA, FAM, FDS RCPS (Glasg)[b],
Anantanarayanan Parameswaran, MDS, DNB, MNAMS, MFDSRCPS, FDSRCS, FFDRCS[c],
Takahiro Kanno, DDS, FIBCSOMS, FIBCSOMS-ONC/RECON, PhD[a],*

KEYWORDS

- Genial surgery • Chin augmentation • Chin reduction • Asymmetry correction • Genioplasty
- Orthognathic surgery

KEY POINTS

- Genioplasty is a versatile procedure and is applicable to various case scenarios.
- The technique was described for over 7 decades and evolved with numerous technical modifications.
- Three-dimensional (3D) clinical and cephalometric assessment of the genium relative to the face is an important prerequisite.
- Preoperative planning can be aided by simulation and 3D models to enable fabrication of cutting guides and patient-specific implants to enhance precision.
- Genioplasty is proved to be a standard procedure to address functional issues.

INTRODUCTION

Facial profile is perceived to be associated with attractiveness and intelligence.[1] Among the various attributes that render balance to a face, the genium/chin constitutes an important part that contributes to the facial profiles. The aesthetics of the lower face is greatly determined by the genium,[2,3] which makes reestablishment of the genial morphology vital in corrective facial surgery.[2] It is hence necessary to evaluate the genium objectively on its individual merit, and any discrepancy is addressed accordingly.[4]

Historically, surgical intervention to correct deformities of the genium was carried out only in cases of retrogenia, wherein autograft placement was facilitated through an extraoral submental incision.[2,5] Aufricht and colleagues performed a genial augmentation using osseocartilaginous tissue obtained from reduction of a dorsal nasal hump.[6] The first surgical procedure performed to correct a genial deformity was an advancement genioplasty. Hofer proposed an extraoral approach for a horizontal symphyseal osteotomy in cadavers.[2] Gillies and Millard replicated Hofer's technique in vivo.[7,8] Obwegeser revolutionized the surgery through an intraoral approach.[2] This was performed to correct a retruded chin in a patient with satisfactory dental occlusion, with the aim to minimize resorption and to facilitate contact healing by retaining good bony approximation. Reichenbach and colleagues described an intrusive/impaction genioplasty to bring forth a vertical

[a] Department of Oral and Maxillofacial Surgery, Shimane University Faculty of Medicine, 89-1, Enyacho, Izumo, Shimane 693-0021, Japan; [b] Department of Oral and Maxillofacial Surgery, SRM Dental College and Hospital, Bharathi Salai, Ramapuram, Chennai 600 089, Tamilnadu, India; [c] Department of Oral and Maxillofacial Surgery, Meenakshi Ammal Dental College and Hospital, Alapakkam Main Road, Maduravoyal, Chennai 600 095, Tamilnadu, India
* Corresponding author. Department of Oral and Maxillofacial Surgery, Shimane University, Izumo, Shimane, Japan.
E-mail address: tkanno@med.shimane-u.ac.jp

Oral Maxillofacial Surg Clin N Am 35 (2023) 97–114
https://doi.org/10.1016/j.coms.2022.06.009
1042-3699/23/© 2022 Elsevier Inc. All rights reserved.

reduction in genial height through a superior rotation of the lower segment after a wedge ostectomy.[2] Converse and Smith published a technique to increase the vertical genial height with interposition of an autograft.[9] Genial tapering and shaping to enhance aesthetics and feminization were reported by Ousterhout.[10] Distraction osteogenesis to widen the mental region was also reported.[11,12] Genioplasty is also indicated to improve lip competency and widening the tongue space for airway improvement in patients with obstructive sleep apnea.[13]

This review aims to present an overview of contemporary genioplasty techniques, their applications, and considerations on stability, osteosynthesis, complications, and the future developments.

ASSESSING A PATIENT FOR GENIOPLASTY

Assessment of the chin should include symmetry, vertical dimension and width relative to the overall shape of the face, and the presence of canting involving the inferior border of mandible.[14] Tide and colleagues proposed a concept of Quick Analysis of the Chin, which included parameters such as (i) lip eversion (due to microgenia and deep overbite), (ii) mandibular anterior teeth evaluation and thickness of chin pad (8–11 mm on an average), (iii) depth and height of the labiomental fold, and (iv) dynamic chin pad motion while smiling. A few important clinical assessments and reference lines are described in **Table 1**.

Role of Genioplasty in Contemporary Orthognathic Surgery

The contemporary principles of orthognathic surgery address the cosmetic as well as functional requirements of a patient with skeletal deformity. The osteotomy design and vector of bony movement are determined by the plane in which correction is required.[2] Hence, a thorough understanding of the deformity in all planes is required to arrive at an accurate diagnosis and to establish a pertinent treatment plan.

Genioplasty for correcting sagittal (anteroposterior) deformities

Alloplastic implants are commonly used for addressing an anteroposterior genial deficiency. This provides satisfactory results in cases with discrepancies of 4 to 5 mm. However, larger corrections may represent a substantial underlying orthognathic deformity and mandate planning to include osseous genioplasties with or without surgery of the maxilla or mandible.[18] Osseous genioplasty also demonstrates better soft tissue

Table 1	
Assessment for genioplasty	
Assessment Parameters	**Definition**
E line (Ricketts, 1954)[15]	Measured from pronasale to pogonion; depicts lip position relative to chin and nose (line should cross 2 mm and 4 mm from lower and upper lips, respectively)
S line (Steiner, 1953)	Subnasale to pronasale to soft tissue pogonion; for lip prominence evaluation (0 ± 2 mm from both upper and lower lips)
Legan's angle[15] (Legan and Burstone, 1980)	Angle formed from lines through glabella to subnasale and subnasale to pogonion; angle of facial convexity ($8°–16°$, average of $12°$)
Zero Meridian (Gonzalles-Ulloa, 1968)[16]	Perpendicular line to Frankfurt's plane through nasion; pogonion should coincide with line or be slightly (0 ± 2 mm) behind line, subnasale 8 mm behind to line
Cervicomental angle	Angle between two tangents. First tangent to the neck at sub-cervical junction (lowest point of submental and neck area juncture) and second tangent to submental area (genium to sub-cervical area); normal values in females is $126°$ and in males is $121°$
Riedel line[17]	Associates the most prominent spots on the lower and upper lips with the protuberant point on the genium
Byrd analysis line[17]	Tangent to the upper lip drawn from mid-dorsal region of nose up to chin. Genium should ideally be 3 mm behind the above tangent

contours in comparison with alloplastic implants.[19] Augmentation of the genium with silicone,[20,21] porous polyethylene (Medpore),[22] expanded polytetrafluoroethylene[21,23,24] (currently not used), hydroxyapatite,[25] and mersilene[26,27] has been described in the literature. To prevent dislodgement of the implants, fixation is usually necessary. Although healing after alloplast placement is faster than osseous genioplasty, it is not suitable for three-dimensional (3D) correction of moderate-to-severe genial deformities.[18] Infection, graft rejection, resorption, extrusion, contraction, and lower lip retraction are the documented complications[28] with alloplasts. However, studies that compared alloplastic implants with osseous genioplasty reported no significant resorption or infection of the alloplast in long term. The use of autograft,[29] allogenic bone graft,[30] and fat grafting[31] for chin contour correction has also been described but with limited success. **Table 2** summarizes the various alloplastic materials and their advantages and disadvantages.

Genioplasty allows the chin to be advanced (**Figs. 1** and **2**) or setback (**Figs. 3** and **4**) in the anteroposterior plane. The indications for anteroposterior correction include (1) retruded/protruded genium, (2) lower third deformity, (3) management of obstructive sleep apnea, and (4) as an adjunct to cosmetic procedures such as rhinoplasty and facelifts. Until the 1950s, setback of the chin was the only practiced technique. With the advent of contemporary methods of planning, the role of osseous genioplasty has expanded significantly.

In a clinical situation that requires pure anteroposterior movement, care is taken to ensure a horizontal osteotomy design in the sagittal plane with minimal oblique angulation (**Fig. 5**). This ensures an optimal movement without any unplanned change in the vertical dimension.[2,37] In case of a combined vertical deformity, the osteotomy design may be modified to incorporate an angulation,[38,39] which depends on the vertical change required. Movement along a true horizontal vector would minimally increase the genial height, whereas reduction of the genial height could be achieved using a steep oblique vector of movement. Advancement or setback of the genium may produce bony protuberances/steps at the junction between osteotomized segment and the mandibular corpus. This needs to be adjusted to achieve a smooth jawline and soft tissue contour.[2,40,41] When extreme advancements of 10 mm to 14 mm are required, interpositional grafts may be placed as required.[42]

Genioplasty for correcting vertical (superoinferior) deformities
Management of vertical discrepancies may be performed to increase or reduce the lower facial height. The correction of mild discrepancies in the vertical dimension can be achieved by modifying the vector of movement in the sagittal plane and the osteotomy design as previously described (see **Fig. 5**). However, true changes to the vertical dimension may be achieved by exclusively downgrafting or impacting the chin after osteotomy.

To increase vertical dimension of the chin, an osteotomy is performed to mobilize the genial segment which is then down-grafted and fixed at the preplanned position. A bone graft is interposed to allow bone contact and improve stability (**Fig. 6**). The placement of the graft should be passive to prevent any inadvertent change of the position.[40]

To reduce chin height, two horizontal osteotomy cuts are performed to remove a predetermined amount of intervening bone (**Figs. 7** and **8**). Care is taken to avoid damage to the root apices. Modifications can be incorporated in the osteotomy design to produce forward or backward rotation of the genial tip. Removal of a bone segment that is wider anteriorly would produce anterior rotation of the genial tip, whereas bone removal that is wider posteriorly rotates the tip posteriorly.[40] If the genium seems redundant, as is the case with most patients with vertical excess, a minimal advancement of the genium can be performed to balance the soft tissue profile.[18]

Genioplasty for correcting transverse (mediolateral) deformities
The chin can be narrowed or widened to correct any transverse deformities (**Fig. 9**). Genioplasty for narrowing is a more commonly performed procedure which facilitates a sharp and triangulated appearance of the chin. The osteotomies can also be tailored to address anterior and posterior component deformities.

To narrow the chin, after completion of the horizontal osteotomy, a predetermined amount of bone is removed from the mid-portion of the osteotomized genioplasty segment. The lateral segments are then medialized and fixed in the midline. In cases where widening is required, a straight midline osteotomy is performed to separate the genium in two pieces with placement of a bone graft in between. For a more predictable transverse correction, Reyneke recommended fixation of an osteosynthesis plate on the midline of the genium and to use it as a pivot before bicortical separation.[40]

Genioplasty for asymmetry correction
Asymmetry corrections require meticulous planning to restitute facial and genial midlines[18] (**Fig. 10**). Pre-osteotomy reference markings are

Table 2
Allografts used in genioplasty: advantages versus disadvantages

Material	Advantages	Potential Disadvantages
Silicone (dimethylpolysiloxane)	• For augmentation • Inert in nature[25]	Bone erosion, excessive fibrosis, foreign body reaction, implant migration, fragmentation infection,[25] and button chin appearance[26]
Acrylic (methylmethacrylate)	• Less inflammatory reactions • Can be used with titanium mesh as a scaffold[32]	Brittle, palpable, resorptive effects,[26] and exothermic during setting[33]
Medpore (porous polyethylene)	• User friendly, good adaptation, and moldability • Allows tissue ingrowth,[25] minimal deformation, migration, and infections[34]	May induce granulomatous reactions Requires good soft tissue coverage (compromised in thin skin areas)[25]
Polyamide mesh (organopolymer related to nylon, Supramid)	• Stabilized by fibrous tissue ingrowth • Provides precise facial contour[25]	Fragmentation, resorption, foreign body reaction due to black carbon particles,[25] and degradation by hydrolysis—resulting in progressive bulk loss every year[26,32]
Hard tissue replacement: polymethylmethacrylate merged with poly-2-hydroxyethylmethacrylate coated with calcium hydroxide	• Biocompatible • Hydrophilic • Inhibits microbial growth due to negative surface charging • Osteoconductive • No resorptive/inflammatory effects[25]	Lack of osteoinductive properties[25]
Gore-Tex (expanded polytetrafluoroethylene)	• Minimal fibrous tissue and capsule formation • Moldable and soft[21]	Severe bone erosion/resorption[23]
Proplast I (with carbon fibers), Proplast II (with aluminum oxide), Proplast hydroxyapatite (HA)	• Moldable • Good connective tissue ingrowth into the implant • Biocompatible[35]	Questionable long-term stability,[36] multinucleate giant cell reaction[35]
HA	• Configuration similar to bone • Osteointegration • Biocompatible[25] • Cement form enables placement in any area • Osteoinductive and osteoconductive[21]	Rigidity, needs good soft tissue cover, hard to shape, difficult to fix,[25] decreased shear resistance,[21] brittle (porous type)[36]
Mersilene (polyester fiber)	• Biocompatible • Minimal displacement[27] • Good strength and durability • Good contour adaptation[26]	• Expensive[27] • Requires good soft tissue cover to prevent dehiscence • Possibility of implant migration[26]

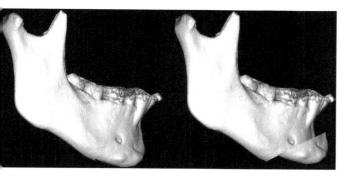

Fig. 1. Advancement genioplasty.

essential to orient the genial segment. A minimum of three reference lines (one midline and two para median) need to be marked perpendicular the osteotomy line. This would facilitate the alignment and synchronization of midlines (facial and genial) during fixation and also provide information regarding the quantum of correction achieved.[40] Chin contouring is an alternative technique to correct asymmetries at the chin region (**Fig. 11**).

Soft tissue changes following genioplasty
Understanding soft tissue changes following skeletal surgery is an important factor to plan postsurgical outcomes. **Table 3** provides a summary of the anticipated soft tissue response to bony chin surgery reported in the literature.

Clinical Application and Effectiveness of Genioplasty for Specific Indications in Maxillofacial Surgery

Obstructive sleep apnea syndrome
Riley and Guilleminault established the use of advancing the genial tubercle along with the genioglossus muscle by genioplasty for the management of obstructive sleep apnea syndrome (OSAS).[47] The investigators performed genial advancement with concomitant surgery to the

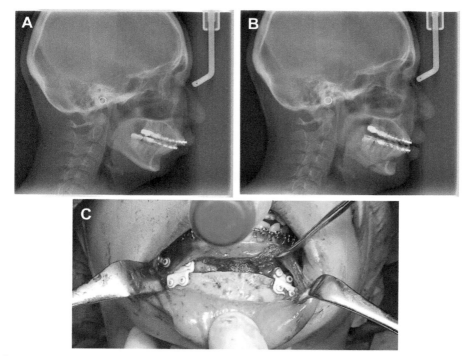

Fig. 2. Advancement genioplasty in a clinical setting. (A) Preoperative cephalogram demonstrating retruded genium. (B) Postoperative cephalogram demonstrating advancement of the genium. (C) Intraoperative picture of advanced segment with fixation.

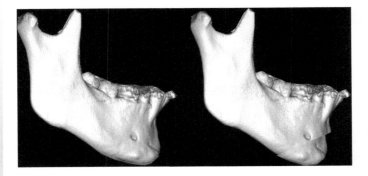

Fig. 3. Setback genioplasty.

hyoid bone. Song and colleagues[48] summarized the advantages of this technique in a meta-analysis: (1) significant reduction in the patients' apneic–hypopneic index apnea-hypopnea index, (2) increase in postoperative oxygen saturation levels, (3) better clinical outcomes when compared with traditional genioplasty alone, and (4) demonstrable advancement of the tongue base anteriorly, with resultant increase in the upper airway space (**Figs. 12** and **13**).

Feminization surgery

Genial sculpting is a vital part of feminization surgeries, which is needed in about 99% of patients. Males tend to have a wider, longer, and more pronounced chin, whereas females feature a soft, oval, or tapering appearance. Minor corrections to the chin can bring considerable changes in the patient's postsurgical appearance. A trapezoidal genial shape can be narrowed by removal of a central bone segment and inferior border ostectomy. A broad genium that conforms a U-shape can be narrowed through a segment resection and inferior border trimming to a V-shape. However, caution should be exercised against over-zealous central fragment removal. In cases of asymmetry, a larger amount of bone removal can be made on the pronounced side.[10] Although every surgery is customized to the patient's needs, some procedures such as shape contouring, prominence removal, and midline ostectomy are empirical.[49] An elaborate analysis of the chin in feminization has been documented by Ousterhout and colleagues.[50] Telang and colleagues summarized facial feminization surgery into three stages: (i) shaving of mandible, gonial angle and Adam's

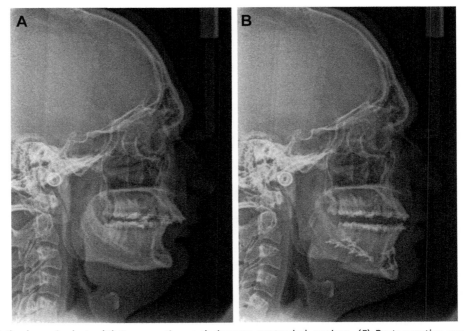

Fig. 4. Setback genioplasty. (*A*) Preoperative cephalogram protruded genium. (*B*) Postoperative cephalogram demonstrating genial setback with fixation.

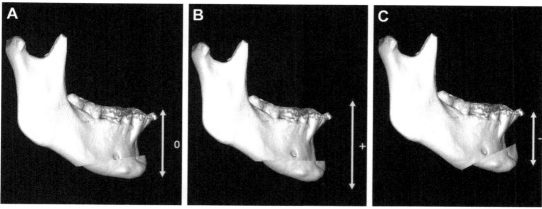

Fig. 5. Influence of osteotomy angulation on the vertical dimension of the lower face. (*A*) Horizontal osteotomy with minimal oblique angulation maintains vertical dimension. (*B*) Pure horizontal movement produces genial elongation. (*C*) Steep oblique osteotomy reduces vertical dimension of the lower face.

apple, (ii) genial reduction and neck lift, and (iii) reconstitution of the upper units (forehead and hairline). The investigators quote that reforming of the lower jaw as well as forehead contouring are among the most preferred procedures.[51]

Residual cleft lip and palate-related deformities

Patients with dentofacial deformities secondary to cleft lip and palate display problems such as decreased upper lip length and/or increased eversion of the lower lip. They may also demonstrate a vertical growth pattern of the mandible with increased vertical height of the lower face. The use of a sliding genioplasty with vertical reduction has been shown to produce an effective relocation of the lower lip and chin soft tissues with improved aesthetic and lip competence.[18] The decision to perform a sliding genioplasty depends on the

clinical indication and can be performed either as the sole procedure or in conjunction with maxillary and/or mandibular procedures.

Functional genioplasty[52] in cleft lip and palate deformities is proven to be successful to regain lip functionality and competence, increase incisor stability, correction of the flat genial contour, and improve esthetics.[52] Subapical osteotomy for management of anterior open bite was put forth by Kole and can be used to manage segment asymmetries.[53] Ramanathan and colleagues have advocated a modification of Kole's procedure in cleft patients with microgenia and open bite deformity, which aimed to maintain the basal bone morphology and vascularity. The group proposed a subapical osteotomy at premolars with an upward positioning, combined with a low-level genioplasty cut and removal of a bony

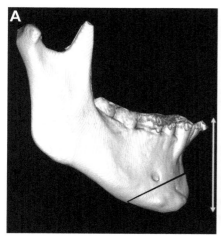
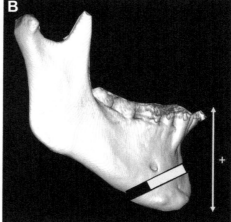

Fig. 6. Vertical augmentation genioplasty for increasing lower facial height. (*A*) Osteotomy design. (*B*) Down-grafting of the lower segment with interpositional bone graft.

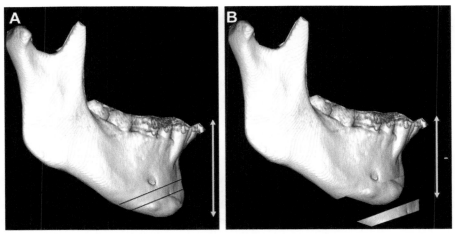

Fig. 7. Vertical reduction genioplasty for reducing lower facial height. (*A*) Osteotomy design demonstrating the segment marked for removal. (*B*) Apposition of osteotomy segments following intermediate ostectomy.

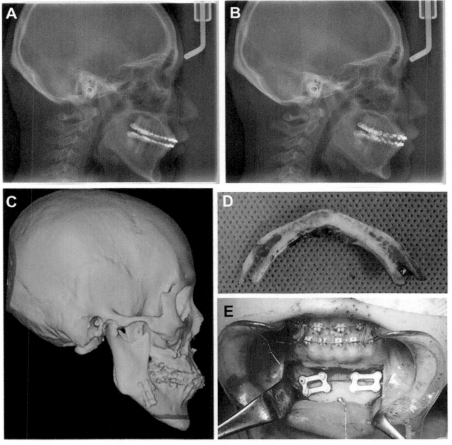

Fig. 8. Vertical reduction genioplasty in a clinical setting. (*A*) Preoperative cephalogram demonstrating vertical genial excess. (*B*) Postoperative cephalogram demonstrating genial reduction. (*C*) Computer-assisted planning for accurate removal of bone. (*D*) Bone removed after ostectomy. (*E*) Fixation of the genial segment after reduction.

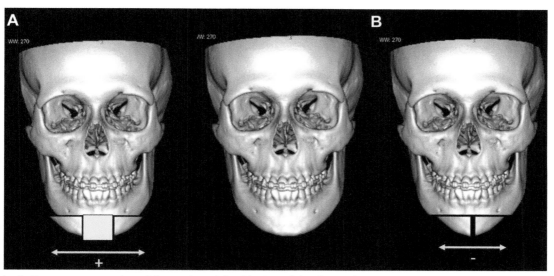

Fig. 9. Transverse correction of the genium. (*A*) Widening of the chin with interpositional bone graft. (*B*) Narrowing of the chin after removal of midline bone.

wedge of 5 mm. The bone wedge was then placed beneath the subapical segment. The investigators have also described to remove the excessive soft tissue at the pogonion through the intraoral access.[54]

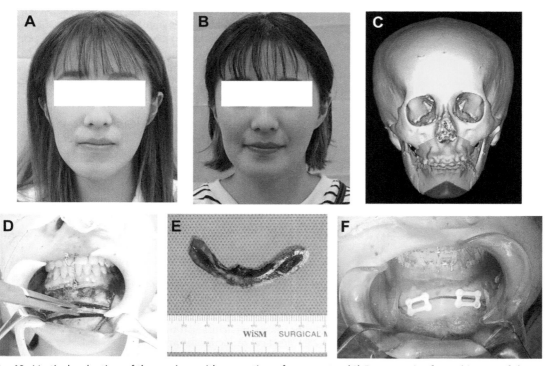

Fig. 10. Vertical reduction of the genium with correction of asymmetry. (*A*) Preoperative frontal image of the patient demonstrating increased lower facial dimension and deviation of the chin to the right side. (*B*) Postoperative frontal image showing correction of the vertical dimension with restitution of skeletal midlines. (*C*) Image demonstrating presurgical plan. (*D*) Ostectomy performed for vertical reduction of the chin. (*E*) Resected bone segment. (*F*) Fixation of the genial segment.

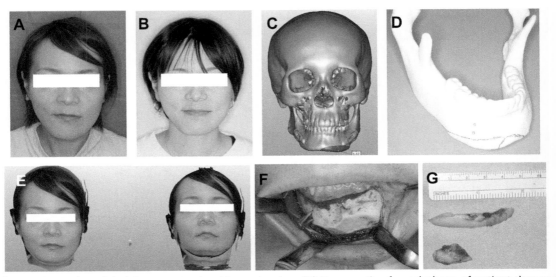

Fig. 11. Correction of facial asymmetry by chin contouring. (*A*) Preoperative frontal photo of patient demonstrating marked asymmetry in the left lower border of the mandible. (*B*) Postoperative frontal photo showing restitution of facial symmetry after lower border contouring. (*C*) Preoperative planning for bone contouring. (*D*) Stereolithographic model depicting areas of interest for bone contouring. (*E*) Three-dimensional planning using photogrammetry for better outcomes. (*F*) Intraoperative image demonstrating bone removal for contouring. (*G*) Bone removed from the lower border.

Osteosynthesis

Historically, wire ligature osteosynthesis was used as nonrigid fixation for genioplasty. However, the use of wires compromises stability, as they allow macro-movement between the fragments. This has paved way for their gradual decline in their clinical use and the development of rigid fixation techniques.

Titanium osteosynthesis

Titanium osteosynthesis may be achieved with screws alone or miniplates with screws. Screw fixation methods involve using lag screw or position screws which are load-sharing[55] and offer good postoperative stability (**Fig. 14**). In screw osteosynthesis, countersinking of the screw head is necessary to prevent palpability and microfractures around the screw head due to induced stresses.[40] It is also important to consider the

---

Table 3
Soft tissue response to genioplasty

Movement/Repositioning Plane	Expected Soft Tissue Change
Advancement	A ratio of soft tissue changes of 0.87:1 is expected[43]
Augmentation	Increased soft tissue advancement results with anterior augmentation.[44] Periosteal stripping of the genial segment can result in soft tissue thinning over the mentum.[45] Alloplastic implantation generates a soft response of 0.8:1[17]
Setback	Soft tissue changes are predicted to be 1:1 but less reliable than advancement. Caution to a "double-chin" appearance
Superior positioning	Vertical repositioning elicits a soft tissue-to-hard tissue ratio change of 0.25:1. Vertical reduction of around 6–8 mm may cause soft tissue redundancy[44] with ptosis
Inferior positioning	A ratio of soft tissue changes of 1:1 is expected
Transverse movements	Soft tissue changes of 71% are reported to bony transverse corrections. With transverse width reduction procedure, soft tissue changes of 0.6:1 are expected[46]

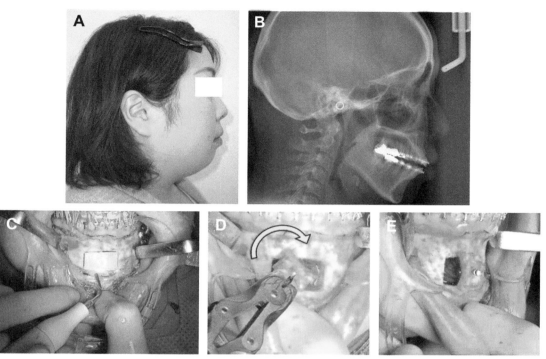

Fig. 12. Genioglossus advancement technique. (*A*) Preoperative profile photograph demonstrating presence of retruded genium and shallow chin throat angle. (*B*) Preoperative lateral cephalogram showing retruded chin and reduced retroglossal airway space. (*C*) Intraoperative image showing marking of the osteotomy window incorporating the genial musculature. (*D*) Advancement of the bony window with the genial muscle attachments. (*E*) Rotation and fixation of the bony window including the advanced genioglossus muscle.

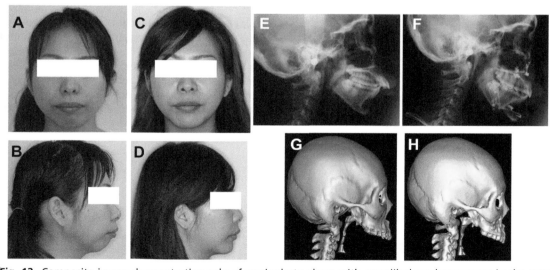

Fig. 13. Composite image demonstrating role of genioplasty along with mandibular advancement in the management of OSAS. (*A*) Preoperative frontal and (*B*) profile demonstrating class 2 skeletal relationship, retruded chin and shallow chin-throat angle. (*C*) Postoperative frontal and (*D*) profile showing excellent soft tissue profile with correction of retrognathia and retrogenia. (*E*) Preoperative and (*F*) postoperative lateral cephalograms demonstrating mandibular and genial advancements for correction of OSAS. (*G*) Preoperative and (*H*) postoperative airway volume rendering demonstrating the absolute increase in retropalatal and retroglossal airway following mandibular and genial advancements.

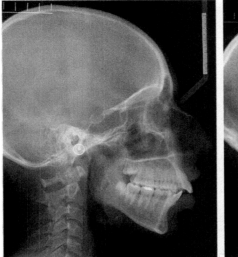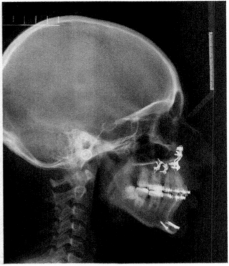

Fig. 14. Radiographs demonstrating osteosynthesis for genioplasty using position screws.

angulation, depth, and direction of the drill and screw to avoid damage to dental roots and the mental nerve.

Osteosynthesis with miniplates and screws[1,37] is the most widely accepted method. Plates are available in various designs including X plate, H plate, and I plate. The availability of prefabricated and pre-bent implants that are specifically designed for genioplasty has made advancements and fixation, easy, and predictable (**Fig. 15**).

Bioresorbable osteosynthesis

Bioresorbable materials have been used and documented for genioplasty with varying degrees of success[56,57] (**Fig. 16**). However, screw head fracture has been a commonly reported complication. Other limitations include increased cost, technique sensitivity, and increased intraoperative time. Also, data on long-term stability concerning biodegradable systems in orthognathic surgery are insufficient.[58–60]

Recent Advances in Computer-Assisted/Aided Surgery for Genioplasty

Technological advances in radiology and computerization in clinical medicine have enabled preoperative virtual planning and simulation for precise osteotomies, repositioning, and fixation for genioplasty (**Fig. 17**). Templates such as cutting guides, fixation guides, and interocclusal 3D printed splints are becoming increasingly popular in orthognathic surgery. These guarantee reduction in intraoperative time and improved accuracy.[18]

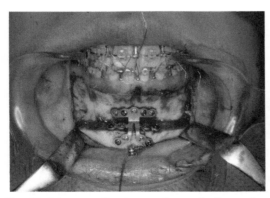

Fig. 15. Intraoperative image demonstrating osteosynthesis for genioplasty using titanium miniplates and screws.

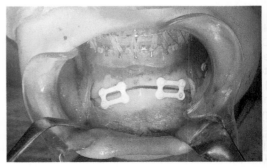

Fig. 16. Intraoperative image demonstrating osteosynthesis for genioplasty using bio-resorbable miniplates and screws.

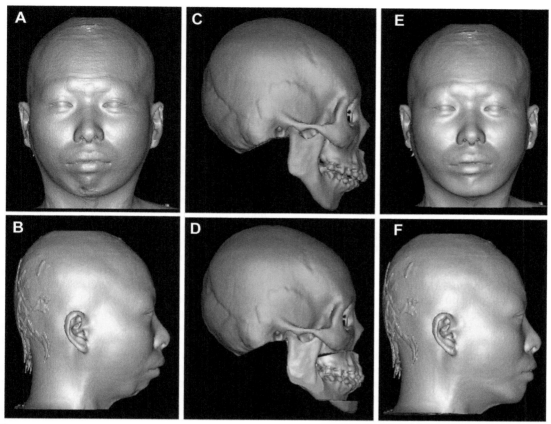

Fig. 17. Composite image demonstrating computer-assisted 3D surgical planning and simulation. (*A*) Preoperative soft tissue moulage frontal and (*B*) profile generated by soft tissue volume rendering. (*C*) Lateral view of patient's skeletal relationship. (*D*) Finalized treatment plan involving bimaxillary surgery and advancement genioplasty. Simulation of treatment plan demonstrating soft tissue changes in the (*E*) frontal and (*F*) profile moulages.

Customized templates for complex genioplasties were traditionally fabricated manually. Assis and colleagues[61] describe the use of acrylic guides for osteotomy and positioning that was fabricated on physical STL (stereolithographic) models for asymmetry correction secondary to TMJ (temporomandibular joint) pathology.

The use of computer-assisted surgery for genioplasty currently uses computer-aided designing (CAD) and computer-aided manufacturing (CAM) technologies with 3D printing for fabrication of stents. The process involves the use of two stents: (i) a cutting guide fabricated for intraoperative use that acts as a tracer for marking the osteotomy line/design and (ii) the positional template that is used to position the segments for final osteosynthesis.[62] These stents can either be bone-borne or tooth-borne depending on the design.[63]

A systematic review published by Oth and colleagues[64] discussed the advantages of CAD/CAM technology for genioplasty. These include (1)

improvement in precision; (2) reduced surgical exposure; (3) preservation of anatomic structures; (4) reduced morbidity; and (5) streamlining of the technique. Significant intraoperative time reduction was observed in two studies which compared conventional with CAD/CAM-executed genioplasty. A study by Li and colleagues[65] compared genioplasty by a tooth-borne guide versus a traditional genioplasty as the control group and concluded that using printed guides effectively decreased intraoperative time and permitted greater accuracy in recreating the surgical plan. Another significant advantage of using 3D planning and guide is the ability to locate and prevent mental nerve injury.

Recent advances in the planning of genioplasty include the technique of genioglossus advancement (osteotomy of the mental segment containing the genioglossus muscle only) for patients with OSAS, with or without genioplasty described by Cheng and colleagues.[66] Favorable results are observed on patients diagnosed with mild-to-moderate

OSAS with this technique. Another innovation was the advocation of a "foundation screw" by Lin and colleagues[67] for correction of facial asymmetry, which proposed the incorporation of a screw head space during planning to guide the final positioning of the osteotomized segment to provide an accurate replication of the presurgical plan.

Complications

Intraoperative
Iatrogenic injuries to the mental nerve may occur due to improper osteotomy technique or presurgical planning, resulting in paraesthesia or anesthesia. If transected, repair of the mental nerve should be performed immediately. The osteotomy should be designed in such a way that the superior cut should be 5 mm inferior to the tooth root of mandibular anterior teeth.[68]

Immediate postoperative
Dehiscence, prolonged pain, edema, infection, lip ptosis, and non-aesthetic outcomes have been reported in literature.[40,69] The incidence of complications arising after a genioplasty is estimated to be less than 5%.[17] Paraesthesia and anesthesia of a transient nature have been reported after the Genial Bone Advancement Trephine method. The complication may be due to excessive traction of the lower lip including the mental nerves.[70]

Late postoperative
Unplanned changes of the osteotomy angulation, relative to the mandibular lower border, may result in unfavorable contour-related changes postoperatively, which could affect the aesthetic outcome and the satisfaction of the patients.[71,72] Excessive muscle detachment from the osteotomized segment may cause soft tissue sag in the mental region and causes lower lip retraction. Improper approximation of the mentalis muscle may also cause ptosis of the lower lip which is characteristically seen as a "witch chin deformity." This can be avoided through realignment of the soft tissues of lips and mentum, and proper layer-wise wound closure with dead space elimination.[73]

Inadequate planning for a sliding genioplasty may produce an "hourglass deformity," that appears as a notch at the inferior border in frontal view. This can be corrected by augmentation with bone grafts 6 months after the initial procedure or by shaving the lateral cortices to achieve a better contour. Another possible complication is a "rippling effect," which can be caused by repositioning of the mentalis too superiorly during lip closure. This may be corrected by re-apposition

of the muscle and skin.[74] In addition, excessive anterior genial advancement can exaggerate the labiomental sulcus (maximal depth: women—4 mm; men—6 mm) and give an aged and unesthetic appearance to the patient. It can be avoided by good presurgical assessment and planning.[17]

Stability

Many studies have highlighted the resorption patterns after an advancement or reduction genioplasty.[75,76] Irrespective of bone remodeling patterns, the shape of the fragment changes over time and becomes smooth. This indicates functional remodeling occurring in the genium after surgery. This remodeling is a result of stress dissipation and changes in muscle equilibrium.[18]

Suprahyoid muscles play a key factor that contributes to the skeletal relapse.[52] This is seen in Tenon–Mortise genioplasty and sliding genioplasty,[77] wherein the muscles do not elongate or stretch.[78,79] Adequate fixation should be used to counteract these muscle forces. Good apposition and bony contact of osteotomized segment should be ensured to reduce skeletal relapse.

Regardless of the method of osteosynthesis, an overall relapse of 8.2% has been observed at the pogonion point after advancement genioplasty, which may be accounted for skeletal instability or bone remodeling.[80,81] Some studies showed that soft tissue stripping caused greater resorption.[76,82] Soft tissue conservation and limited periosteal stripping were known to promote neovascularization, decrease bone mass loss and enhance stability.[83] Bone in adolescents demonstrate a greater degree of resorption than adult.[84] It is recommended that osteosynthesis should generally be avoided in areas of resorption to improve stability in the long term.[80]

FUTURE PERSPECTIVES

The constant endeavor in clinical research is to create a safer and efficient surgical environment for the patient while ensuring better outcomes and quality of life. Minimally invasive incisions as advocated by Van Roy and colleagues and Nadjmi and colleagues may be options to minimize postsurgical bony resorption in the genial segments while improving stability.[85,86] The use of piezosurgery and ultrasonic scalpel systems has also enhanced surgical ease and reduced blood loss while selectively protecting vital neurovascular tissues. This may very well become a routine in the future with more efficient bone cutting equipment. Oth and colleagues described a technique of less invasive genioplasty that employed the use of piezosurgery combined with 3D planning and 3D-printed templates to promote postoperative healing and reduce surgical time and complication rates.[64] Robotic surgeries are now being performed increasingly across the world. With the advent of 3D techniques, genioplasty using robots can be considered a viable alternative in the near future.[87]

SUMMARY

This article discusses the utility of genioplasty in contemporary orthognathic surgery with an overview of techniques, their indications, and applications to address various clinical scenarios. Recent advances with the use of CAD/CAM technology have further improved the accuracy and safety for genioplasty as a useful orthognathic procedure.

CLINICS CARE POINTS

- Angulation of osteotomy design is important and influences the vertical dimension of the lower third of the face.
- Position of the mentolabial fold influences the outcome after genioplasty. A low mentolabial fold accentuates the chin, whereas a high mentolabial fold accentuates the entire lower face.
- Genioplasty is a versatile procedure and plays an important role in the surgical management of obstructive sleep apnea and facial feminization surgery.
- Understanding soft tissue changes for genioplasty is paramount in achieving optimal esthetics.

DISCLOSURE

This work was in part supported by JSPS KAKENHI Grant Number - 21K10042 to T. Kanno. M. Ramanathan: Data collection, manuscript writing. E. Panneerselvam: Critical analysis and input, manuscript editing. A. Parameswaran: Critical analysis and input, manuscript editing. T. Kanno: Critical analysis and input, manuscript editing.

REFERENCES

1. Sinko K, Jagsch R, Benes B, et al. Facial aesthetics and the assignment of personality traits before and after orthognathic surgery. Int J Oral Maxillofac Surg 2012;41(4):469–76.

2. da-Silva H, Marinho L, Souza G, et al. About Chin (Genioplasty) Surgery. Int J Morphol 2020;38(4): 1120–7.

3. Lee TS, Kim HY, Kim TH, et al. Contouring of the lower face by a novel method of narrowing and lengthening genioplasty. Plast Reconstr Surg 2014; 133(3):274e–82e.

4. Mani V. Orthognathic Surgery for Mandible. In: Bonanthaya K, Panneerselvam E, Manuel S, et al, editors. Oral and maxillofacial surgery for the clinician. 1st edition. Singapore: Springer; 2021. p. 1477–512.

5. Steinhäuser EW. Historical development of orthognathic surgery. J Craniomaxillofac Surg 1996;24(4): 195–204.

6. Aufricht G. Combined nasal plastic and chin plastic. Am J Surg 1934;25(2):292–6.

7. Miles B, Leach J. Osseous genioplasty: Technical considerations. Oper Tech Otolaryngol Head Neck Surg 2007;18(3):181–8.

8. San Miguel Moragas J, Oth O, Büttner M, et al. A systematic review on soft-to-hard tissue ratios in orthognathic surgery part II: Chin procedures. J Craniomaxillofac Surg 2015;43(8):1530–40.

9. Converse JM, Wood-Smith D. Horizontal osteotomy of the mandible. Plast Reconstr Surg 1964;34:464–71.

10. Park S, Noh JH. Importance of the chin in lower facial contour: narrowing genioplasty to achieve a feminine and slim lower face. Plast Reconstr Surg 2008;122(1):261–8.

11. Epker BN, Fish LV, editors. Dentofacial deformities: integrated orthodontic and surgical correction. St. Louis: Mosby; 1995. p. 507.

12. Raoul G, Wojcik T, Ferri J. Outcome of mandibular symphyseal distraction osteogenesis with bone-borne devices. J Craniofac Surg 2009;20(2):488–93.

13. Schendel SA. Genioplasty: a physiological approach. Ann Plast Surg 1985;14(6):506–14.

14. Reyneke J. Systematic Patient Evaluation. In: Essentials of orthognathic surgery. China: Quintessance; 2003. p. 13–68.

15. Arroyo HH, Olivetti IP, Lima LF, et al. Clinical evaluation for chin augmentation: literature review and algorithm proposal. Braz J Otorhinolaryngol 2016; 82(5):596–601.

16. Naini FB, Garagiola U, Wertheim D. Analysing chin prominence in relation to the lower lip: The lower lip-chin prominence angle. J Craniomaxillofac Surg 2019;47(8):1310–6.

17. Baker SB. Genioplasty. In: Weinzweig J, editor. Plastic surgery secrets plus. 2nd edition. Philadelphia: Mosby Elsevier; 2010. p. 573–8.

18. Gupta RJ, Precious DS, Schendel SA. Genioplasty. In: Fonseca R. Oral and maxillofacial surgery. 3rd edition. China: Elsevier; 2018. p. 96–112.

19. Mohammad S, Dwivedi CD, Singh RK, et al. Medpore versus osseous augmentation in genioplasty procedure: A comparison. Natl J Maxillofac Surg 2010;1(1):1–5.

20. Aynehchi BB, Burstein DH, Parhiscar A, et al. Vertical incision intraoral silicone chin augmentation. Otolaryngol Head Neck Surg 2012;146(4): 553–9.

21. Friedman C, Costantino P. Alloplastic materials for facial skeletal augmentation. Facial Plast Surg Clin North Am 2002;10(3):325–33.

22. Rojas YA, Sinnott C, Colasante C, et al. Facial Implants: Controversies and Criticism. A Comprehensive Review of the Current Literature. Plast Reconstr Surg 2018;142(4):991–9.

23. Shi L, Zhang ZY, Tang XJ. Severe bone resorption in expanded polytetrafluoroethylene chin augmentation. J Craniofac Surg 2013;24(5): 1711–2.

24. Harris WC, Raggio BS. In: StatPearls, editor. Facial chin augmentation. 2021. Available at: https://www. ncbi.nlm.nih.gov/books/NBK554506/ 2021.

25. Ziccardi V, Johns F, Demas P, et al. Current alloplastic materials in augmentation genioplasty. Am J Cosmet Surg 1997;14(1):55–61.

26. Gross EJ, Hamilton MM, Ackermann K, et al. Mersilene mesh chin augmentation. a 14-year experience. Arch Facial Plast Surg 1999;1(3):183–90.

27. Fariña R, Valladares S, Aguilar L, et al. M-shaped genioplasty: a new surgical technique for sagittal and vertical chin augmentation: three case reports. J Oral Maxillofac Surg 2012;70(5):1177–82.

28. Chang EW, Lam SM, Karen M, et al. Sliding genioplasty for correction of chin abnormalities. Arch Facial Plast Surg 2001;3(1):8–15.

29. Tang X, Gui L, Zhang Z. Analysis of chin augmentation with autologous bone grafts harvested from the mandibular angle. Aesthet Surg J 2009;29(1):2–5.

30. Posnick JC, Sami A. Is it safe and effective to lengthen a chin with interpositional allogenic (Iliac) graft? J Oral Maxillofac Surg 2015;73(8): 1583–91.

31. Rohrich RJ, Sanniec K, Afrooz PN. Autologous fat grafting to the chin: a useful adjunct in complete aesthetic facial rejuvenation. Plast Reconstr Surg 2018;142(4):921–5.

32. Quatela VC, Chow J. Synthetic facial implants. Facial Plast Surg Clin North Am 2008;16(1):1–v.

33. Rubin JP, Yaremchuk MJ. Complications and toxicities of implantable biomaterials used in facial reconstructive and aesthetic surgery: a comprehensive review of the literature. Plast Reconstr Surg 1997; 100(5):1336–53.

34. Gui L, Huang L, Zhang Z. Genioplasty and chin augmentation with Medpore implants: a report of 650 cases. Aesthetic Plast Surg 2008;32(2): 220–6.

35. Parkes ML, Kamer FM, Merrin ML. Proplast chin augmentation. Laryngoscope 1976;86(12):1829–35.

36. Karras SC, Wolford LM. Augmentation genioplasty with hard tissue replacement implants. J Oral Maxillofac Surg 1998;56(5):549–52.

37. Ferretti C, Reyneke JP. Genioplasty Atlas Oral Maxillofac Surg Clin North Am 2016;24(1):79–85.

38. Yang DB, Park CG. Mandibular contouring surgery for purely aesthetic reasons. Aesthetic Plast Surg 1991;15(1):53–60.

39. Dolce C, Johnson PD, Van Sickels JE, et al. Maintenance of soft tissue changes after rigid versus wire fixation for mandibular advancement, with and without genioplasty. Oral Surg Oral Med Oral Pathol Oral Radiol Endod 2001;92(2):142–9.

40. Reyneke J. Surgical Technique. In: Essentials of orthognathic surgery. China: Quintessance; 2003. p. 247–307.

41. Hinds EC, Kent JN. Genioplasty: the versatility of horizontal osteotomy. J Oral Surg 1969;27(9):690–700.

42. Salyer KE, Xu H, Portnof JE, et al. Skeletal facial balance and harmony in the cleft patient: Principles and techniques in orthognathic surgery. Indian J Plast Surg 2009;42:S149–67.

43. Talebzadeh N, Pogrel MA. Long-term hard and soft tissue relapse rate after genioplasty. Oral Surg Oral Med Oral Pathol Oral Radiol Endod 2001; 91(2):153–6.

44. Gallagher DM, Bell WH, Storum KA. Soft tissue changes associated with advancement genioplasty performed concomitantly with superior repositioning of the maxilla. J Oral Maxillofac Surg 1984;42(4): 238–42.

45. Bell W, Proffit W, White R. Surgical correction of dentofacial deformities. Philadelphia: Saunders; 1980.

46. Segner D, Höltje WJ. Langzeitergebnisse nach Genioplastik [Long-term results after genioplasty]. Fortschr Kieferorthop 1991;52(5):282–8.

47. Riley R, Guilleminault C, Powell N, et al. Mandibular osteotomy and hyoid bone advancement for obstructive sleep apnea: a case report. Sleep 1984;7(1):79–82.

48. Song SA, Chang ET, Certal V, et al. Genial tubercle advancement and genioplasty for obstructive sleep apnea: A systematic review and meta-analysis. Laryngoscope 2017;127(4):984–92.

49. Deschamps-Braly J. Feminization of the Chin: Genioplasty Using Osteotomies. Facial Plast Surg Clin North Am 2019;27(2):243–50.

50. Ousterhout DK. Feminization of the chin: a review of 485 consecutive cases. Bologna, Italy: Medimond International Proceedings; 2003. p. 10.

51. Telang PS. Facial Feminization Surgery: A Review of 220 Consecutive Patients. Indian J Plast Surg 2020; 53(2):244–53.

52. Precious DS, Delaire J. Correction of anterior mandibular vertical excess: the functional

genioplasty. Oral Surg Oral Med Oral Pathol 1985; 59(3):229–35.

53. Kole H. Surgical operations on the alveolar ridge to correct occlusal abnormalities. Oral Surg Oral Med Oral Pathol 1959;12(3).

54. Ramanathan M, Rao SH. A Modified Kole's Osteotomy for Correction of Anterior Open Bite and Macrogenia in a Cleft Patient. Craniomaxillofac Trauma Reconstr 2013;6(1):57–60.

55. Reyneke JP, Johnston T, van der Linden WJ. Screw osteosynthesis compared with wire osteosynthesis in advancement genioplasty: a retrospective study of skeletal stability. Br J Oral Maxillofac Surg 1997; 35(5):352–6.

56. Park YW. Bioabsorbable osteofixation for orthognathic surgery. Maxillofac Plast Reconstr Surg 2015;37(1):6.

57. Kanno T, Sukegawa S, Furuki Y, et al. Overview of innovative advances in bioresorbable plate systems for oral and maxillofacial surgery. Jpn Dent Sci Rev 2018;54(3):127–38.

58. Edwards RC, Kiely KD, Eppley BL. Resorbable fixation techniques for genioplasty. J Oral Maxillofac Surg 2000;58(3):269–72.

59. Bhatt K, Roychoudhury A, Bhutia O, et al. Equivalence randomized controlled trial of bioresorbable versus titanium miniplates in treatment of mandibular fracture: a pilot study. J Oral Maxillofac Surg 2010;68(8):1842–8.

60. Salvino MJ. Avoiding pitfalls in craniofacial reconstruction using absorbable plates. J Craniofac Surg 2010;21(1):213–4.

61. Assis A, Olate S, Asprino L, et al. Osteotomy and osteosynthesis in complex segmental genioplasty with double surgical guide. Int J Clin Exp Med 2014;7(5): 1197–203.

62. Yamaguchi K, Lonic D, Lo LJ. Complications following orthognathic surgery for patients with cleft lip/palate: A systematic review. J Formos Med Assoc 2016;115(4):269–77.

63. Wang LD, Ma W, Fu S, et al. Design and manufacture of dental-supported surgical guide for genioplasty. J Dent Sci 2021;16(1):417–23.

64. Oth O, Orellana MF, Glineur R. The Minimally Invasive-Guided Genioplasty Technique using Piezosurgery and 3D printed surgical guide: An innovative technique. Ann Maxillofac Surg 2020;10(1):178–81.

65. Li B, Wei H, Zeng F, et al. Application of a novel three-dimensional printing genioplasty template system and its clinical validation: a control study. Sci Rep 2017;7(1):5431.

66. Cheng A. Genioglossus and genioplasty advancement. Atlas Oral Maxillofac Surg Clin North Am 2019;27(1):23–8.

67. Lin S, Hsiao Y, Chang C, et al. Osseous Genioplasty with the use of a "Foundation Screw". Glob Surg 2017;3(1):1–4.

68. Wang J, Gui L, Xu Q, et al. The sagittal curving osteotomy: a modified technique for advancement genioplasty. J Plast Reconstr Aesthet Surg 2007; 60(2):119–24.

69. Lindquist CC, Obeid G. Complications of genioplasty done alone or in combination with sagittal split-ramus osteotomy. Oral Surg Oral Med Oral Pathol 1988;66(1):13–6.

70. Miller FR, Watson D, Boseley M. The role of the Genial Bone Advancement Trephine system in conjunction with uvulopalatopharyngoplasty in the multilevel management of obstructive sleep apnea. Otolaryngol Head Neck Surg 2004; 130(1):73–9.

71. Schuberth G, Shaughnessy T, Timmis D. Mandibular advancement and reduction genioplasty. Am J Orthod Dentofacial Orthop 1990;98(6):481–7.

72. Shoshani Y, Chaushu G, Taicher S. The influence of the osteotomy slope on bony changes after advancement genioplasty. J Oral Maxillofac Surg 1998;56(8):919–23.

73. Olate S, Zaror C, Blythe JN, et al. A systematic review of soft-to-hard tissue ratios in orthognathic surgery. Part III: Double jaw surgery procedures. J Craniomaxillofac Surg 2016;44(10): 1599–606.

74. Dennis T, Bains A, Doumpiotis D. Correction of a genioplasty. Br J Oral Maxillofac Surg 2019;57(5): 481–2.

75. McDonnell JP, McNeill RW, West RA. Advancement genioplasty: a retrospective cephalometric analysis of osseous and soft tissue changes. J Oral Surg 1977;35(8):640–7.

76. Ellis E 3rd, Dechow PC, McNamara JA Jr, et al. Advancement genioplasty with and without soft tissue pedicle: An experimental investigation. J Oral Maxillofac Surg 1984;42(10):637–45.

77. Wiese KG. Extreme Kinnvorverlagerung mit der Tandemgenioplastik [Extreme chin advancement with tandem genioplasty]. Mund Kiefer Gesichtschir 1997;S1:S105–7.

78. LaBanc JP, Epker BN. Changes of the hyoid bone and tongue following advancement of the mandible. Oral Surg Oral Med Oral Pathol 1984;57:351.

79. Ellis E III, Carlson DS. Stability two years after mandibular advancement with and without suprahyoid myotomy: an experimental study. J Oral Maxillofac Surg 1983;41:426.

80. Precious DS, Cardoso AB, Cardoso MC, et al. Cost comparison of genioplasty: when indicated, wire osteosynthesis is more cost effective than plate and screw fixation. Oral Maxillofac Surg 2014;18(4): 439–44.

81. Shaughnessy S, Mobarak KA, Høgevold HE, et al. Long-term skeletal and soft-tissue responses after advancement genioplasty. Am J Orthod Dentofacial Orthop 2006;130(1):8–17.

82. Polido WD, de Clairefont Regis L, Bell WH. Bone resorption, stability, and soft-tissue changes following large chin advancements. J Oral Maxillofac Surg 1991;49(3):251–6.

83. Storum KA, Bell WH, Nagura H. Microangiographic and histologic evaluation of revascularization and healing after genioplasty by osteotomy of the inferior border of the mandible. J Oral Maxillofac Surg 1988; 46(3):210–6.

84. Tulasne JF. The overlapping bone flap genioplasty. J Craniomaxillofac Surg 1987;15(4):214–21.

85. Van Roy S, Nadjmi N, Van Hemelen G, et al. A new minimally invasive genioplasty procedure. Int J Oral Maxillofac Surg 2017;46:169.

86. Nadjmi N, Van Roy S, Van de Casteele E. Minimally Invasive Genioplasty Procedure. Plast Reconstr Surg Glob Open 2017;5(11):e1575.

87. Lim SH, Kim MK, Kang SH. Genioplasty using a simple CAD/CAM (computer-aided design and computer-aided manufacturing) surgical guide. Maxillofac Plast Reconstr Surg 2015;37(1):44.

Rhinoplasty as an Adjunct to Orthognathic Surgery: A Review

Tian Ee Seah, BDS (Singapore), MDS (OMS, Singapore), FRACDS (Aus), FAMS (Singapore), Director[a,b,*], Velupillai Ilankovan, FRCS (Edin & Eng), FDSRCS (Edin & Eng)[c]

KEYWORDS

- Concurrent • Septorhinoplasty • Septoplasty • Turbinoplasty • Rhinoplasty • Orthognathic surgery
- Maxillary osteotomy • Lefort I osteotomy

KEY POINTS

- The aim of simultaneous rhinoplasty and orthognathic surgery is to correct both dentofacial deformities and nasal deformities of the patients.
- Nasal deformities include inherent nasal deformities or surgically induced nasal changes.
- Challenges exist in assessing the nose accurately postmaxillary osteotomy due to surgical edema and temporary distortion of the nose from nasal intubation.
- Simultaneous rhinoplasty and orthognathic surgery can be carried out for patients with a high degree of satisfaction as it is a single operation, general anesthesia, and postoperative healing.
- Staged rhinoplasty can be performed for cases in which the surgeon feels that simultaneous rhinoplasty is not suitable.

INTRODUCTION

Orthognathic surgery (OGS) is an established and recognized method to correct dentofacial deformities.[1] One of the goals of OGS is to exhibit improved soft tissue change, reflecting the optimal correction of the maxilla and mandible. This positive soft tissue change is the result of improved midface support, paranasal areas, nasolabial angles, and proportion of upper lip to lower lip contours. Ultimately, there is a significant improvement in the patient's postoperative facial profile, esthetics, and function.

The nose is integral to the face. In OGS, particularly maxillary surgeries, the nose plays a critical role in determining its final nasal esthetics. The Le Fort I osteotomy is the most frequently performed maxillary osteotomy in orthognathic surgeries. Soft tissue changes to the nose which are attributed to the maxillary movements have been

well documented.[1–4] Depending on the pre-existing nasal characteristics, these acquired effects can be favorable or unfavorable.

Unfavorable nasal results can happen despite careful planning and execution in placing the maxillomandibular structures in their correct relationship. Such undesirable nasal effects can eclipse the positive results from the bony correction and can be upsetting to both the patient and surgeon. This is more so when the preoperative nasal characteristics seemed to be favorable before the OGS.

NASAL CHANGES FROM MAXILLARY MOVEMENT

Widening of the alar base is a common sequela of Le Fort I osteotomy because it entails circumvestibular subperiosteal dissection, an incision that causes the release and splaying of the facial musculature from

[a] TES Clinic for Face and Jaw; [b] Kadang Kerbau Women and Children's Hospital, National Dental Centre Singapore, Singapore General Hospital, Changi General Hospital; [c] Department of Maxillofacial/ Head and Neck Surgery, University Hospitals Dorset NHS Foundation Trust, Dorset, United Kingdom
* Corresponding author. 304 Orchard Road, Lucky Plaza Medical Suites #05-42, Singapore 238863.
E-mail address: stianee@yahoo.com

Oral Maxillofacial Surg Clin N Am 35 (2023) 115–126
https://doi.org/10.1016/j.coms.2022.06.008
1042-3699/23/© 2022 Elsevier Inc. All rights reserved.

the underlying bone.[2] There are several documented methods to reduce this effect, including nasal cinch,[3,4] V-Y closure,[4,5] or preservation of the anterior nasal spine.[2]

Other surgically induced changes in the nose are mostly vector-dependent. Maxillary impaction can cause superior positioning of the nasal tip; alar widening; retraction of the columella at the subnasal region; as well as a decrease in the nasolabial angle. Maxillary advancement can cause cephalic rotation of the nasal tip; increased supratip depression; and shortening of the nasal tip and alar widening.[1,6] The resulting effect is an increased nostril shown with a widened and shortened nose. Maxillary down graft can cause inferior repositioning of the alar base and columella. A maxillary setback can cause droopy nasal tip lobule with decreased support for the nasal tip.[1,2]

Nasal morphology and deformities should be carefully recorded during a clinical examination. It is important to take photographic records, including frontal, profile, oblique views; worm's view and bird's eye view. Where indicated, a computed tomographic (CT) scan, cone-beam computer tomography scan, or a nasoendoscopy should be carried out.

Nasal deformities can be classified into (1) inherent nasal deformities that can be improved by OGS, (2) inherent nasal deformities that cannot be improved by OGS, and (3) nasal characteristics and deformities that can be worsened by OGS.

Nasal Deformities that Will be Improved by Orthognathic Surgery

There are nasal deformities that can be improved by maxillary surgery. Maxillary advancement and impaction can improve patients with mild nasal hump; droopy or ptotic nasal tip or a narrow alar base.[1,4]

Although maxillary advancement can cause a corresponding decrease in the nasal tip height, its superior rotation can improve the ptotic nasal tip and improve the profile of the nose. This is because the cephalic rotation of the nasal tip can result in (1) straightening of the nasal bridge in patients with a mild dorsal hump or (2) reducing the prominence of a mild nasal hump. Increased maxillary support at the piriform region from maxillary impaction and advancement can also result in widened alar width and this can be advantageous for patients with narrow alar bases. In patients presenting with maxillary asymmetry and corresponding septal deviation, correction of the maxilla asymmetry restores the anterior nasal spine to the midline. A mildly deviated septum can be

corrected by releasing the perichondrium of the septal mucosa before the disjunction of the septal cartilage and vomer. Fixing the nasal septum to the corrected anterior nasal spine can improve the deviation. These corrections can be done via the Le Fort I approach.

Nasal Deformities that Will NOT be Improved by Orthognathic Surgery

Some nasal deformities cannot be improved by OGS. These are nasal deformities that will remain unchanged although the effects of the vector of the maxillary movement do not cause untoward effects on the nose.

These include nasal and severe septal deviations; wide nasal bridges; flat or shallow nasal dorsum; moderate to prominent dorsal hump; bifid or flat amorphous nasal tip; wide alar bases; and upturned noses with increased nostril show.[1,2]

Nasal Characteristics and Deformities that Will be Worsened by Orthognathic Surgery

Maxillary advancement is indicated for patients with moderate to severe maxillary hypoplasia. These patients may not present with nasal deformities but may, as a consequence of increased paranasal bony support from large maxillary movements, end up with a less esthetic nasal result. Large maxillary advancements will result in an increased cephalic rotation of the nose with increased nostril show and accentuation of the supratip break. There is also a corresponding decrease in nasal tip height as the nose splays laterally. The nasal bridge can also look comparatively shallower with large advancements.

Nasal deformities, such as a flat or shallow nasal dorsum; bulbous, amorphous nasal tip; wide alar bases; and upturned noses with increased nostril show can potentially look worse after large maxillary impactions and advancement because of the earlier mentioned reasons.

These include nasal deformities arising in syndromic patients, such as cleft lip and palate patients. These patients usually have unchanged or worsened nasal deformities due to large maxillary advancement.

In patients with moderate or large prominent dorsal hump, the dorsal hump may look more prominent with maxillary setbacks. Similarly, patients with the droopy nasal tip will lose further bony support in maxillary setbacks and down grafts resulting in a more ptotic nasal tip.

THE CASE FOR SIMULTANEOUS RHINOPLASTY AND ORTHOGNATHIC SURGERY

Seah and colleagues[1] retrospectively studied 75 Caucasian patients and found that 61% of the patients had mild to prominent cosmetic nasal abnormalities, whereas 19% of the patients had genial deformities. Despite the greater prevalence of patients with nasal deformities than chin deformities, they found that it was common to correct the chin simultaneously but not the nose. With the nose sitting at the prominent part of the face, the authors felt that it was ideal for the nose to be corrected concurrently to achieve a better facial profile and appearance. They suggested that simultaneous rhinoplasty and OGS should be considered for two groups of patients: (1) those with inherent nasal deformities and (2) those who acquired surgically induced nasal deformities from the OGS. They performed nine cases of simultaneous rhinoplasty and orthognathic over a year and found that there were no functional or esthetic complications.

In 1988, Waite and colleagues[4] published a case series of patients who underwent 22 septorhinoplasties and concurrent orthognathic surgeries. Among these patients, 15 cases were with concurrent bimaxillary osteotomies and 7 with isolated bilateral sagittal split osteotomies. The patients were followed up for at least 12 months. Among these patients, they found that 82% of their patients were pleased with their rhinoplasty results, whereas 94% of their patients were pleased with their jaw surgery. Further, 84% would recommend having both surgeries together, whereas 16% would consider a staged nasal surgery.

Waite and colleagues[4] found that rhinoplasty can compensate for unfavorable nasal changes from maxillary procedures. They suggested that patient selection is important for simultaneous rhinoplasty. They also considered patients to be suitable candidates for concurrent surgeries if (1) they have an average noticeable nasal problem and (2) have a reasonable understanding and expectations of the improvement. Other relative indications include morphologic deformities, such as (3) functional nasal septal deviations or deviations that have no significant functional issues. (4) Minor tip defects, such as an excessive amorphous or bulbous tip, can undergo simultaneous tip-plasty, whereas (5) prominent dorsal hump can be straightened or reduced concurrently.[7]

Raffaini and colleagues[2] have the largest cohort to date involving 250 patients who underwent bimaxillary osteotomies and concurrent rhinoplasty over a 1-year period. Like Seah and colleagues, they were also in favor of simultaneous correction of nasal deformities that remain relatively unchanged after OGS, as well as acquired nasal deformities. The authors acknowledged the challenges that existed in assessing the nose accurately after bimaxillary surgery and showed that these could be surmounted by both meticulous preoperative planning. In their large group of patients, all the patients were found to have good functional and esthetic outcomes. Their study found that 94% of the patients felt that they accepted rhinoplasty only because it was included in the single operation together with OGS strengthening the case for concurrent nasal and dentofacial corrections. This was in line with the findings of Waite and colleagues.

Posnick and colleagues[8] studied patients who underwent bimaxillary osteotomies, septoplasties, and turbinoplasties and found an overall satisfaction rate of 95%.

Costa and colleagues[9] performed simultaneous rhinoplasty, bimaxillary osteotomies, and functional endoscopic sinus surgery on 13 patients. They noted that the advent of rigid fixation had allowed concurrent rhinoplasty and OGS because it allowed the safe transfer of the nasal to oral intubation while limiting surgical relapse alluding to one of Waite and colleagues' observations.[4] In their study, they found that all the patients had good esthetic and functional results and were free of previous rhinosinusitis.

Sun and Steinbacher[10] retrospectively studied a group of 68 orthognathic patients who underwent staged or simultaneous rhinoplasty. Among this cohort of patients, 12 patients underwent simultaneous rhinoplasty with OGS of which 2 underwent bimaxillary osteotomies and 10 had mandibular surgeries. They reported patient satisfaction in the surgical results in both staged and simultaneous groups with no revisions needed at 1.5 years of follow-up.

Besides nonsyndromic patients, the paper by Kinnebrew and Emison in 1987 included patients with a plethora of syndromes showing that concurrent correction of nasal and skeletal structures can be done for this group of patients[11] Some of these patients had Binder's syndrome, Sainton syndrome, Saethre–Chotzen syndrome, and cleft lip and palate syndrome. Another case study by Seah[12] reported on the feasibility of correcting both the nasal deformity and jaw deformity on a cleft lip and palate patient who underwent bimaxillary osteotomies, genioplasty, and open septorhinoplasty in a single operation.

The advantages of simultaneous rhinoplasty and OGS include a single planning procedure and general anesthesia and postoperative recovery.[13] Infraorbital nerve temporary hypoesthesia, due to the Le Fort I procedure can also make recovery more comfortable for the patient.

SURGICAL APPROACHES

The choice of surgical approaches to the nose is often dependent on the type of nasal deformity to be corrected. The common approaches are closed rhinoplasty or open rhinoplasty.[1,2,4]

Closed rhinoplasty has been reported for correction of isolated dorsal hump reduction or mild saddle nose augmentation during simultaneous rhinoplasty and OGS.[2,4] This involves marginal or infracartilaginous incisions or intercartilaginous incisions. Intercartilaginous can gain direct access to the nasal bridge, whereas marginal or infracartilaginous approaches can gain access to the nasal tip as well as the dorsum. For an infracartilaginous incision, it can be further joined to a hemitransfixion incision to give improved surgical access. Alternatively, a separate hemitransfixion or Killian incision can be placed to give access to the septum if septoplasty is required. The benefit of closed rhinoplasty is the absence of a columellar scar, but the challenges include limited surgical exposure.

The open rhinoplasty method is preferred by some surgeons if tip refinement work is required. Raffaini and colleagues[2] reported in their retrospective study that 95% underwent the open rhinoplasty approach. Open rhinoplasty can be performed using an inverted-V, step incision, or V-incision at the narrowest width of the columella with extensions to marginal incisions. This allows excellent visualization of the nasal tip and the dorsum and is useful for complex refinement of the nasal tip. Its drawback is the presence of a columellar scar although this can be minimized with careful and meticulous closure.

The facial degloving approach is the third approach described by Kinnebew and Emision.[11] This approach was first published by Egyedi in 1974[14] and involves degloving the nose via circumferential intranasal incisions with sharp dissection on the subcutaneous plane over the alar cartilage rims. Dissection can be carried out in a subperiosteal plane to the nasofrontal region superiorly and maxilla laterally, which allows visualization of the nose, the maxilla, and the infraorbital rims.[15] Despite the improved visibility, authors cautioned against using this approach for mild nasal deformities because of the possibility of nasal stenosis attributed to the 360° incisions in the vestibular region. This can contribute to issues with tip definition as well asymmetric nares.[11]

SEPTOPLASTY AND TURBINOPLASTY

Septal deviation correction can be done via the Le Fort I approach after the down-fracture of the maxilla. This prevents another endonasal mucosal incision.[4] Seah and colleagues.[1] found that maxillary down-fracture allowed easier access to the septum.

Alternatively, the septal deviation can be addressed during septorhinoplasty either via an endonasal septal mucosal approach using hemitransfixion or Killian incisions or through an open rhinoplasty approach via a split-tip technique. In removing the deviated part of the septum, important considerations should be given to preserving at least 10 mm of the caudal and dorsal strut. The resected deviated septum can be further utilized as cartilaginous grafts. With regards to cases with severe septal deviation requiring subtotal cartilage reconstruction, some surgeons prefer to stage the procedure 6 months after the OGS.[2]

Turbinoplasty is not rhinoplasty per se but is part of nasal surgery and helps with improving the nasal airway in patients with hypertrophic inferior turbinates. Enlarged turbinates can be approached after the down-fracture of the maxilla. The nasal mucosa can be incised to gain access to the inferior turbinates, which can be partially resected. In the author's experience, hemostasis is better controlled when the mucosa of the tubinates as well as the nasal mucosa are sutured with a running 5/0 or 4/0 vicryl suture on a round needle.

MANAGEMENT OF DORSAL DEFORMITIES

Problems of the dorsum are likely because of height discrepancies or deviation of the dorsum.

Deviated Nose

Deviation of the nose can be corrected simultaneously with the correction of dentofacial deformity. The deviation may be because of the cartilaginous vault or the nasal bone. In cases where the deviation is the cartilaginous vault, the septum has invariably deviated and it may suffice to perform septoplasty. The use of spreader or septal extended grafts can further aid in its correction. If the maxilla has deviated, then correction of the maxilla will bring the anterior nasal spline (ANS) to the correct position. The inferior caudal septum can then be anchored to the ANS just before the maxillary mucosal closure.

When the nasal bony vault has also deviated, lateral and medial nasal bone osteotomies can be done with either an endonasal method or percutaneous method, or a combination of both. Care must be given to the maxillary bone plates and the osteotomes should not encroach on the plates (**Figs. 1–8**).

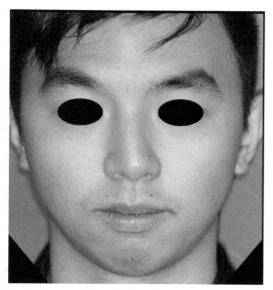

Fig. 1. Preoperative photo of a male patient with skeletal II relationship, maxillary cant and facial asymmetry, and a deviated nose (frontal view).

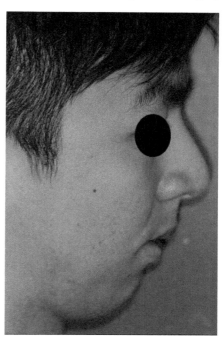

Fig. 3. Preoperative photo of a male patient showing deviated nose (bird's eye view). Preoperative photo of same male patient with hypoplastic mandible and retrogenia (profile view)

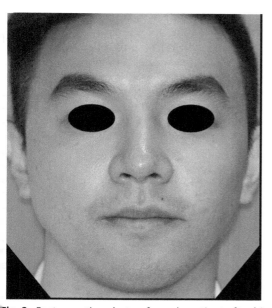

Fig. 2. Postoperative photo of a male patient after bimaxillary osteotomy, advancement genioplasty, and simultaneous open septorhinoplasty, including septal extended graft, columellar strut, onlay grafts, and medial and lateral nasal osteotomy. Improved facial proportions and facial symmetry and improved nasal symmetry (frontal view).

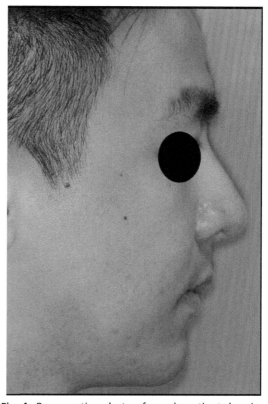

Fig. 4. Preoperative photo of a male patient showing deviated nose (worm's view). Postoperative photo of a male patient showing improved facial profile (profile view)

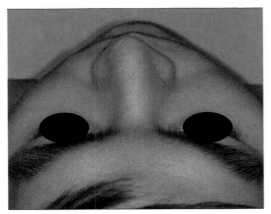

Fig. 5. Preoperative photo of a male patient showing deviated nose (bird's eye view).

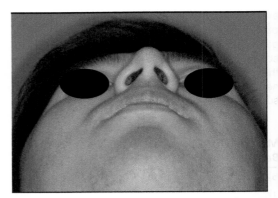

Fig. 7. Preoperative photo of a male patient showing deviated nose (worm's view).

Hump Reduction

In patients with high dorsum, simultaneous hump reduction can be performed. This can be carried either via closed or open rhinoplasty. Hump reduction can be carried out using an incision through the cartilaginous part to be resected followed by osteotomy using Rubin osteotome. After the appropriate reduction, a nasal rasp is used to smoothen the irregularities at the dorsum. When performed simultaneously with OGS, it is preferable to under-correct than to over-correct. Firstly, advancement and impaction of the maxilla can cause cephalic rotation of the nasal tip, which can make the dorsal hump less prominent thus requiring less reduction. Secondly, if tip-plasty is planned to increase nasal tip projection, then this should be taken into consideration when reducing the height of the dorsum. The reason is that the combination of excessive dorsal reduction and increased nasal tip projection can result in an accentuated supratip break.

Dorsal Augmentation

There is a dearth of papers that describe simultaneous dorsal augmentation and OGS in patients with shallow dorsum. Kinnebrew and Emison treated eight patients with dorsal augmentation using onlay graft to the nasal dorsum. Among these patients, seven patients used bone harvested from the iliac bone crest, whereas one patient had Proplast II (Vitek Corp, Houston) placed at the dorsum.[11] Waite and colleagues[7]. also described a patient who had a rib graft to augment the dorsum via infracartilaginous and transfixion approach.

Augmentation materials can include autogenous grafts, such as septal, conchal, and costochondral cartilage.[16] Alloplastic materials, such as silicone[16,17] or Gore-Tex (expanded polyfluoroethylene)[18,19] had been described in rhinoplasties and are popular in Asia. Augmentation of the dorsum can be safely carried out by using autogenous grafts or alloplastic materials with success in rhinoplasty. Although silicone and expanded polyflouroethylene's use in simultaneous rhinoplasty

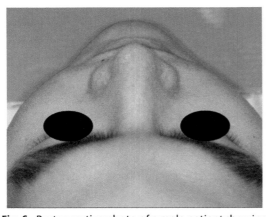

Fig. 6. Postoperative photo of a male patient showing correction of deviated nose (bird's eye view).

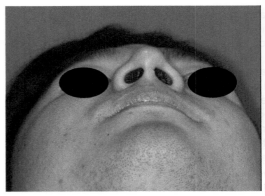

Fig. 8. Postoperative photo of a male patient showing symmetry of the nasal nares after septorhinoplasty (worm's view).

and OGS have not been described before, this is partly attributed to an absence of papers with regard to simultaneous rhinoplasty and orthognathic surgeries in Asian patients. The author has used these materials for dorsal augmentation in simultaneous rhinoplasty and orthognathic surgeries with success (**Figs. 9–14**).

MANAGEMENT OF NASAL TIP DEFORMITIES
Boxy Nasal Tip and Droopy Nasal Tip

Patients with a boxy nasal tip can undergo cephalic trim of the lower lateral cartilage to help reduce the boxiness. Patients with bifid tips will benefit from the placement of crushed cartilage in the interdomal region. Mild droopy nasal tip may be corrected by the advancement of the maxilla. However, if the nasal tip remains droopy, the cephalic trim of the lower lateral cartilage can help to rotate the nasal tip further in the cephalic direction.

Nasal Tip that has Inadequate Projection

Tip-plasty in the form of supratip or lobule grafts using cartilage and Proplast (polytetra-fluoroethylene) had been performed by Kinnebrew and Emison.[11]

In patients with a flat nasal tip with inadequate projection, projection of the nasal tip can be gained by using a septal extension graft and columellar strut to increase the nasal tip projection. The septal extension graft, first described by Bryd and colleagues.[20] is a powerful method to increase nasal tip projection or to derotate the nasal tip. Further reinforcement of the projecting structure can be done by the use of columellar struts.[18] This sits between the lower lateral cartilage and the superior end is fixed to the medial crus of the lower lateral cartilages and the septal extension graft. The inferior end sits superior to the anterior nasal spine. Kinnebrew and Emison described the use of columellar struts using autogenous bone and cartilage when necessary.

If further tip definition and more projection of the nasal tip lobule are required, onlay grafts can be placed in the interdomal region. The authors secure these to the underlying lower lateral cartilages with 5/0 polydioxanone sutures These onlay grafts can be layered if the height is inadequate. Most of the time, conchal grafts or septal grafts are used for these purposes. The authors find that conchal grafts are particularly suitable for this area because it has a natural convex shape and forms the ideal nasal tip projection. Shield grafts can be further used to reinforce columellar struts and structural supports (**Figs. 15–20**).

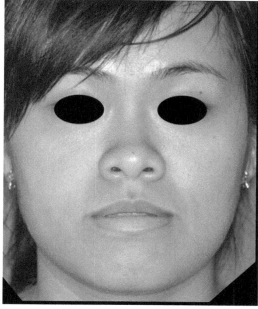

Fig. 9. Preoperative frontal photo of a female patient with skeletal III relationship showing a flat and upturned nose with wide alar base (frontal view).

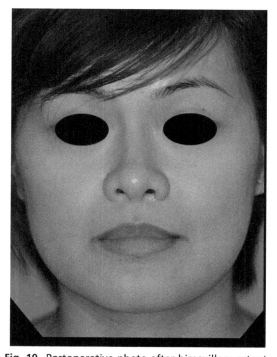

Fig. 10. Postoperative photo after bimaxillary osteotomy and simultaneous open septorhinoplasty, including septal extended graft, columellar strut, and layered onlay grafts at the nasal tip. Dorsum is augmented with Gore-Tex (expanded polytetrafluoroethylene). Alar base reduction (frontal view).

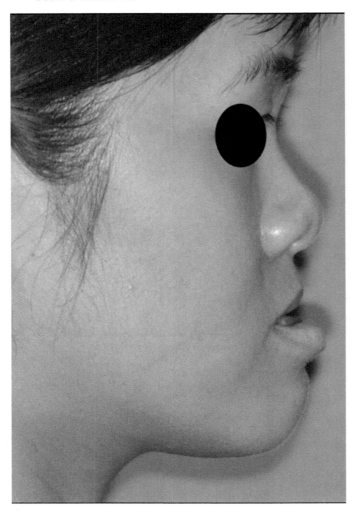

Fig. 11. Preoperative photo of same female patient with maxillary hypoplasia and mandibular hyperplasia. Saddle nose with short upturned nasal tip (profile view).

ALAR BASE DEFORMITIES

The alar base reduction can be carried out in two ways. In the first method, wedge excision or weir reduction can be done by carefully excising the alar rims and suturing them. The incision should be close to the alar crease for good scar formation. In the second method, alar base sills are excised in a diamond or trapezoidal shape at the vestibule of the nostrils to reduce the alar base. In the third method, a combination of wedge and sill excision can be done.

CHALLENGES AND LIMITATIONS TO SIMULTANEOUS RHINOPLASTY AND ORTHOGNATHIC SURGERY

Seah and colleagues.[1] classified challenges in simultaneous rhinoplasty with OGS under preoperative, perioperative, and postoperative considerations.

Preoperative planning is more challenging because the surgeon will need to predict the nasal changes arising from the maxillary movement. The surgeon thus has to be cognizant of these nasal changes with respect to the vector of the maxillary movement and may have to correct not only the inherent nasal deformities but also these nasal changes.

Perioperatively, challenges include surgically induced edema around the nose and paranasal regions, which makes an assessment of the post-maxillary osteotomy nose more difficult. Temporary minor nasal changes may also occur because of the pull of the nasotracheal tube. The surgeons will need to rely on their preoperative planning and not be distracted by the perioperative swelling or nasal distortion. Intraoperatively tube change from nasoendotracheal to oroendotracheal will require an experienced anaesthetist.

Postoperatively, nasal packs are usually placed postsurgically to reduce bleeding and prevent the

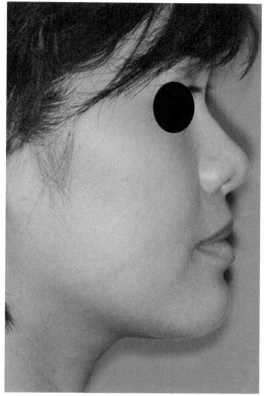

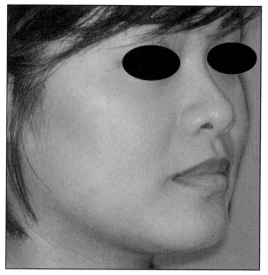

Fig. 14. Postoperative photo of a patient showing improved facial contours and improved dorsal height, nasal tip position, and reduced alar base and acceptable alar base scar (oblique view).

Fig. 12. Postoperative photo of a patient showing improved maxillomandibular relationship and improved dorsal height, nasal tip projection, and position (profile view).

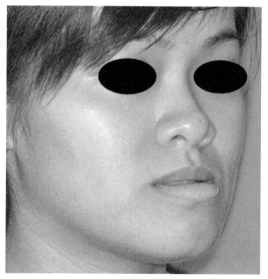

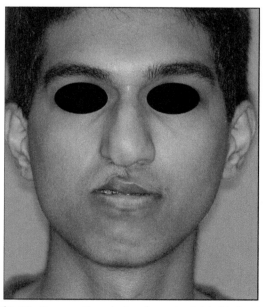

Fig. 13. Preoperative photo of a female patient showing concave facial contours, incompetent lips, shallow dorsum, wide alar base, and upturned nose (oblique view)

Fig. 15. Preoperative photo of a male right-sided unilateral repaired cleft lip and palate with maxillary hypoplasia and nasal asymmetry and bifid nasal tip (frontal view).

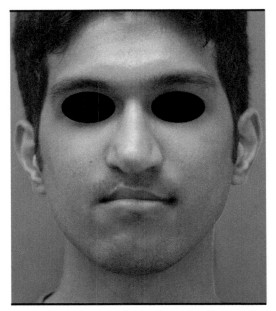

Fig. 16. Postoperative photo of a male after maxillary advancement and simultaneous open septorhinoplasty and right alar rim repositioning showing improved midface support and improved nasal symmetry and obliteration of bifid nasal tip (frontal view).

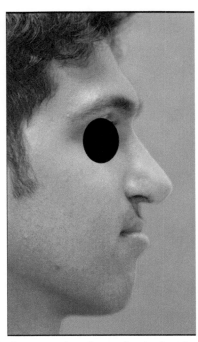

Fig. 18. Postoperative photo after Le Fort I advancement and open septorhinoplasty, including dorsal hump reduction, lateral nasal bone osteotomy, septal extension graft, columellar strut, and layered onlay grafts. Improved facial and nasal profile (profile view).

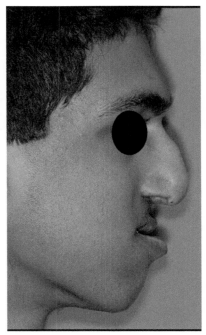

Fig. 17. Preoperative photo of same unilateral right-sided repaired cleft lip and palate patient with skeletal III relationship, prominent dorsal hump, and droopy nasal tip.(profile view).

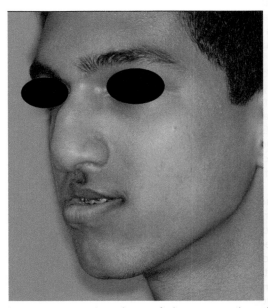

Fig. 19. Preoperative photo of the same unilateral right-sided repaired cleft lip and palate patient showing midface hypoplasia with prominent dorsal hump and incompetent lips (oblique view).

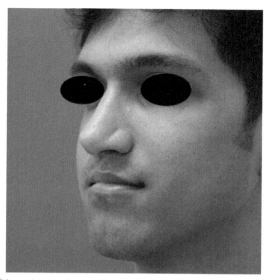

Fig. 20. Postoperative photo of patient with improved facial contours, straight dorsum, improved nasal tip position, and competent lips after simultaneous maxillary advancement and open septorhinoplasty (oblique view).

formation of hematoma, particularly at the septum. Hence, there is also a need for rigid or semi-rigid fixation because training elastics or elastic intermaxillary fixation can only be placed only after the nasal pack is removed; usually on the second postoperative day. In the rare event when unfavorable fractures occur during the osteotomies and intermaxillary fixation is indicated, rhinoplasty will have to be deferred. In such instances, rhinoplasty is usually staged as a second procedure 6 months later.

After the surgery, the patient may complain about periorbital swelling and ecchymosis caused by the rhinoplasty and nasal obstruction because of crusting of the dried mucus along the nasal passage. Placement of the external nasal splint may also be affected by maxillary edema. The use of Doyle splints post-rhinoplasty can be more comfortable for the patients and allow some form of nasal breathing.

Raffaini and colleagues described some contraindications to simultaneous rhinoplasty and orthognathic surgeries. Patients with major functional problems due to severe septal deviation, requiring subtotal cartilage reconstruction are contraindicated for simultaneous corrections. Staged rhinoplasty is also indicated when an unpredictable final occlusion is achieved during OGS. Finally, excessive intraoperative bleeding; compromised rigid fixation; and compromised airways preclude simultaneous nasal procedures. Most papers agree that staged rhinoplasty should be usually delayed at least 6 months.[2,10,21]

THE CASE FOR STAGED RHINOPLASTY AS AN ADJUNCT TO ORTHOGNATHIC SURGERY

Waite and colleagues.[4] recommended staging the rhinoplasty for complex maxillary osteotomies or in instances when the soft tissue cannot be predicted. They suggested avoiding treating extremes in the form of very mild and prominent nasal deformities and suggested that these should be staged.

Sun and Steinbacher[10] also looked at 56 patients who underwent staged rhinoplasty after OGS. In this retrospective study, they were more inclined to perform staged rhinoplasty in situations where (1) maxillary advancement is more than 5 mm; (2) there is more than 2 mm impaction, and if, (3) alar base reduction is indicated. Sun and Steinbacher also preferred to stage rhinoplasty for surgically induced nasal deformities and described a comprehensive list of techniques in the treatment of these different surgically induced deformities.[10]

COMPLICATIONS AND RISKS

Raffaini and colleagues found that the complication rate for nasal surgeries performed with Le Fort 1 ostetomy was 9.2% (23 patients), which was comparable to complications that arose from isolated primary rhinoplasty (6%). Complications included a single complication or a combination of complications. These included nasal dorsum irregularities; residual nasal septum deformities; nasal tip deformities; persistent respiratory limitations; and internal nasal valve collapse. The 23 patients subsequently underwent successful revision rhinoplasty for their deformities.[2]

Waite and Matukas noted in their paper that revision after simultaneous rhinoplasty should not be viewed as a failure as primary rhinoplasty frequently requires further modification.[7]

SUMMARY

The nose is an important consideration in OGS. It can be adversely affected by certain vectors during maxillary osteotomies. Proper case selection, knowledge of OGS, and the nasal changes that accompany various maxillary vectors are important. In-depth knowledge of various rhinoplasty techniques is paramount to correct specific nasal problems: inherent or acquired.

Simultaneous rhinoplasty and orthognathic surgeries have been published in various papers and have been proven to be viable solutions for patients who exhibit both problems. The advantages of simultaneous rhinoplasty and OGS include a single planning procedure and general anesthesia and postoperative recovery.[21] Infraorbital nerve temporary hypoesthesia due to the Le Fort I procedure can also make recovery more comfortable for the patient. The most gratifying advantage of simultaneous rhinoplasty and OGS lies in the dramatic improvement of the patient's overall esthetics and function in a single operation.

In cases where concurrent rhinoplastic surgery is not suitable, the surgeon can stage it 6 months after the OGS. Revision of the nose after simultaneous or staged rhinoplasty should not be viewed as a failure because primary rhinoplasty frequently requires revision to achieve perfection.

CLINICS CARE POINTS

- It is important to examine the nasal morphology of the nose during the orthognathic planning and predict the possible nasal changes that will arise from the planned maxillary vector.
- There are some nasal characteristics that will be improved after maxillary surgery and rhinoplasty is not required for these patients.
- Nasal deformities that will not be improved or can be worsened by the maxillary surgery should be recognized and correction for these deformities should be planned.
- The surgeon should be cognizant of the unfavorable esthetic changes to the nose arising from certain large maxillary vectors, such as impaction or advancement and plan for its correction.
- There are various rhinoplasty techniques that can be used to treat various nasal deformities and the surgeon should be familiar with them.

DISCLOSURE

The author has nothing to disclose.

REFERENCES

1. Seah TE, Bellis H, Ilankovan V. Orthognathic patients with nasal deformities: case for simultaneous orthognathic surgery and rhinoplasty. Br J Oral Maxillofac Surg 2012;50:55–9.
2. Raffaini M, Cocconi R, Spinelli G, et al. Simultaneous Rhinoseptoplasty and Orthognathic Surgery: Outcome Analysis of 250 Consecutive Patients Using a Modified Le Fort I Osteotomy Aesthetic. Plast Surg 2018;42:1090–100.
3. Loh FC. A new technique of alar base cinching following maxillary osteotomy. Int J Adult Orthodon Orthognath Surg 1993;8:33–6.
4. Waite PD, Matukas VJ, Sarver DM. Simultaneous rhinoplasty procedures in orthognathic surgery. Int J Oral Maxillofac Surg 1988;17:298–302.
5. Muradin MSM, Rosenberg AJWP, van der Bilt A, et al. The influence of a Le Fort I impaction and advancement osteotomy on smile using a modified alar cinch suture and V-Y closure: a prospective study. Int J Oral Maxillofac Surg 2012;41:547–52.
6. Mitchell C, Oeltjen J, Panthaki Z, et al. Nasolabial Aesthetics. J Craniofac Surg 2007;18:756–65.
7. Waite PD, Matukas VJ. Indications for simultaneous orthognathic and septorhinoplastic surgery. J Oral Maxillofac Surg 1991;49:133–40.
8. Posnick JC, Wallace J. Complex orthognathic surgery: Assessment of patient satisfaction. J Oral Maxillofac Surg 2008;66:934.
9. Costa F, Salvo I, Sembronio S. Simultaneous functional endoscopic sinus surgery and esthetic rhinoplasty in orthognathic patients. J Oral Maxillofac Surg 2008;66:1370–7.
10. Sun AH, Steinbacher DM. Orthognathic surgery and rhinoplasty: simultaneous or staged? Plast Reconstr Surg 2018;141:322–9.
11. Kinnebrew MC, Emison JW. Simultaneous maxillary and nasal reconstruction. An analysis of twenty-five cases. J Craniomaxillofac Surg 1987;15:312–25.
12. Seah TE. Simultaneous Orthognathic Surgery and Rhinoplasty for the Repaired Unilateral Cleft Lip and Palate Patient: A Case Report. Proc Singapore Healthc 2014;23:191–5.
13. Cottrel DA, Wolford LM. Factors influencing combined orthognathic and rhinoplastic surgeries. Int J Adult Orthodon Orthognath Surg 1993;8:265–76.
14. Egyedi P. Degloving the nose. J Maxillofac Surg 1974;2:101.
15. Kinnebrew MC, Zide MF, Kent JN. Modified LeFort I procedure for simultaneous correction of maxillary and nasal deformities. J Oral Maxillofac Surg 1983; 41:295–304.
16. Malone M, Pearlman S. Dorsal augmentation in rhinoplasty: A survey and review 2015;31(3):289–94.
17. Kim IS. Augmentation rhinoplasty using silicone implants. Facial Plast Surg Clin North Am 2018;26:285–93.
18. Li D, An Y, Yang X. An overview of Asian rhinoplasty. Ann Plast Surg 2016;77(suppl 1):S22–4.
19. Godin MS, Waldman SR, Johnson CM. Nasal augmentation using Gore-Tex. Arch Facial Plast Surg 1999;1:118.
20. Bryd HS, Burt JD, Andochick S, et al. Septal extension grafts: a method for controlling tip projection and shape. Plas Reconstr Surg 1997;100:999.
21. Tan MH, Seah TE, Goh BT. Staged orthodontic, orthognathic surgery and open septorhinoplasty for management of Cleidocranial Dysplasia: A case report. Sci Rep 2020;3:3–4.

Definitive Rhinoplasty and Orthognathic Surgery for Patients with Cleft Lip Palate

Riham Eldesouky, MD, Amir Elbarbary, MD*

KEYWORDS

- Cleft nasal deformity • Definitive cleft rhinoplasty • Cleft orthognathic

KEY POINTS

- All patients with a cleft lip deformity have an associated nasal deformity that ranges in severity.
- Cleft patients present with common anatomic differences, such as a maxilla deficiency in all 3 axes, that arise from intrinsic factors and because of previous surgery.
- Analysis and performance of orthognathic surgery should be conducted before definitive cleft rhinoplasty to optimize the overall result.
- A thorough understanding of the anatomy of the cleft nose aids the surgeon in selecting proper techniques for repair.
- When dealing with cleft patients, surgical technique must be altered in terms of the planned incision.
- Goals of definitive rhinoplasty include relief of nasal obstruction, creation of symmetry, and definition of the nasal base and tip, and management of nasal scarring and webbing.
- Septal reconstruction in the cleft nose is a key maneuver in cleft rhinoplasty.
- The surgeon must be able to use multiple treatment modalities to address the cleft patient and minimize relapse.

INTRODUCTION

Patients with clefts lip and/or palate require long-term multidisciplinary care to achieve functional occlusion and aesthetic facial balance. Because of the existing substantial asymmetry and insufficiency of underlying soft tissue and bone, the nasal deformity associated with congenital cleft lip/palate is a complicated condition that causes major aesthetic and functional challenges.[1] Cleft patients have typical anatomic skeletal anomalies including bony deficits along the premaxilla and the pyriform rim[2] as well as the shortage of the maxilla in all 3 axes, which are caused by both inherent causes and influenced by surgical interventions.[3] To maximize the overall result, definitive cleft rhinoplasty should be evaluated for and performed following underlying skeletal correction. This may require orthognathic surgery to correct skeletal discrepancies. The purpose of this article is to review definitive rhinoplasty and orthognathic procedures in the treatment of patients with cleft lip and palate.

Anatomy and Pathophysiology of the Cleft Nasal Deformity

Nasal deformity exists in all forms of cleft lip with or without cleft palate. The degree of nasal deformity parallels the severity of labial clefting and is also worse whenever associated with clefting of the alveolus and secondary palate. Some common features of the cleft lip nasal deformity have been described.[4] While long-term follow-up studies documented better outcomes and reduced complexity of operative maneuvers required during definitive rhinoplasty when primary "tip rhinoplasty" was performed at the time of unilateral[5]

Department of Plastic, Burns, and Maxillofacial Surgery, Ain-Shams University, Cairo, 11591, Egypt
* Corresponding author.
E-mail address: amir_elbarbary@med.asu.edu.eg

Oral Maxillofacial Surg Clin N Am 35 (2023) 127–137
https://doi.org/10.1016/j.coms.2022.06.011
1042-3699/23/© 2022 Elsevier Inc. All rights reserved.

and bilateral[6] cleft lip repairs, it has been advised to conduct definitive rhinoplasty to correct secondary cleft lip nasal deformity after orthognathic correction and defer further intervention while the nose is still growing and changing rapidly until late childhood and young adulthood, especially for minor and moderate nasal deformities.[7]

Unilateral cleft nasal deformity

The orbicularis oris insertion points are disturbed when there is a unilateral cleft. The orbicularis oris muscle joins to the ipsilateral aspect of the columella on the noncleft side and pulls the premaxilla, columella, and caudal nasal septum to the unaffected side. The orbicularis oris inserts into the ipsilateral alar base and pushes it laterally, inferiorly, and posteriorly on the cleft side. The cleft side's lower lateral cartilage (LLC) is frequently deformed, contributing to the nasal deformity by providing a more blunted contour. Because of blunted medial crus and enlarged lateral crus, the cleft side's nostril is much larger and laterally positioned to the unaffected side (**Fig. 1**A–C). Pathogenesis of the cleft lip nasal deformity is partly the result of an extrinsic factor caused by the misdirected pull of the muscle and also due to an intrinsic deficiency of the alar cartilage that makes it prone to the deformational forces by the mal-inserted perinasal and orbicularis oris muscle.[8]

The nasal septum deviates toward the cleft side as the caudal septum deviates toward the unaffected side. Nasal obstruction is increased when there is a septal deviation and a narrowed nasal aperture. Internal vestibular webbing along the cleft side's nose margin causes the margin to shift inward. Because the LLC is turned inward, the external nasal valve collapses, causing more nasal blockage.[9]

Bilateral cleft nasal deformity

The existence of a bilateral hypoplastic maxilla with no nasal floor development is a notable observation in these patients. The alar base is caudally and laterally positioned, with substantial broadening. Because the lateral crus has grown longer and the medial crus has shrunk, the nasal tip has lost projection and contour. The presence of vestibular webbing can be seen on both sides. The nasal septum is normally near the middle of the nose, contributing to its symmetry (**Fig. 2** A–C). In asymmetric cases the less affected side exerts a pushing strain on the septum, causing septal deviation to the ipsilateral side.[9,10]

Secondary and acquired nasal deformity

Secondary cleft lip nasal deformity is defined as those distortions that persist despite primary operative maneuvers and are expressed as the combination of residual deformity, iatrogenic deformity, and growth-related nasal distortion.[9] Residual deformity is a result of failure to correct, undercorrect, or relapse and is influenced by a variety of factors including the embryologic deficiencies of both the nose and underlying maxillary segments, and the diminished growth potential. Iatrogenic deformities are determined by the pattern of repair of the mal-inserted perinasal and orbicularis oris muscle at the time of primary surgery of the lip, the unintended results of surgical technical errors, and the level of orthodontics practiced within the overall management. Growth-related nasal distortions, also referred to as postsurgical growth potential, occur during puberty and are often worse in children with unilateral cleft lip with or without cleft palate.[9,11,12]

Facial Skeleton Characteristics of Patients with Clefts

Cleft patients are commonly present with a hypoplastic maxilla and a constricted maxillary dental arch.[13](**Fig. 3**: a–d and 4: a–c). On the other hand, unrepaired cleft patients have been reported to develop fairly normal maxillary growth. These observations directed many craniofacial surgeons to believe that multiple surgical interventions at an early age led to subsequent scar formation of contracture and were attributed as the sole cause of hypoplasia.[14]

The severity of maxillary hypoplasia is related to the cleft type.[15] In unilateral cases, the lesser maxillary segment is most commonly hypoplastic and is displaced superiorly, posteriorly, and medially. The maxillary midline is commonly deviated toward the side of the cleft. Bilateral cleft cases tend to present with an extremely narrow maxilla that results from the posterior alveolar segments collapsing medially. This can be seen clinically as a bilateral posterior cross-bite. The premaxilla may be either superiorly or inferiorly positioned and is often protruded.[16] Patients with bilateral CL/P seeking orthognathic surgery notably suffer from multiple residual problems, such as scarring, agenesis of lateral incisors, alveolar defects, abnormal nasal anatomy, and upper lip muscular dysfunction.[17]

SURGICAL MANAGEMENT
Preorthognathic Consideration

Orthodontic preparation

Orthodontics can be used to align and improve the location of the maxillary segments before alveolar bone grafting (ABG). Maxillary expansion is accomplished with the use of fixed

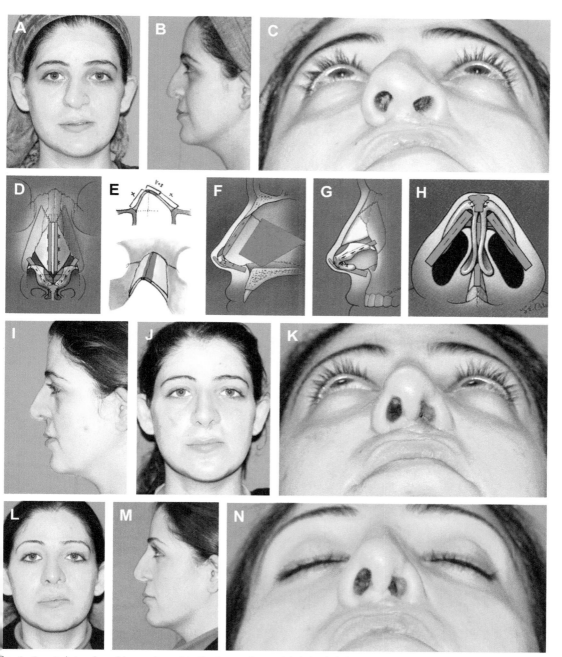

Fig. 1. Front, lateral and base views (*A–C*) of a patient with left cleft lip nasal deformity demonstrating typical features of this type of nose dysmorphology. Her rhinoplasty (*D–H*) consisted of asymmetric osteotomies, asymmetric bilateral spreader grafts, columellar strut graft, release of left lower lateral cartilage with bilateral alar strut, and a shield graft through an open approach. Six weeks (*I–K*) and 2 years (*L–N*) postoperative front, oblique, and base views. (*From* Ince B, Dadaci M. Base Nasal Bone Resection versus Oblique Nasal Bone Resection: A comparative Study of the Outcomes for the Deviated Nose. Plast Reconstr Surg. 2017;139(1):29e-37e. (see **Fig. 1E**))

rthodontic appliances and expanders.[3] Orthodontic treatment continues following ABG or scheduled to be completed when the patient reaches skeletal maturity in preparation for orthognathic surgery. The concept of surgery-first approach is seldom adopted in treatment protocols for cleft patients.[3] The teeth closest to the cleft should be upright with excellent

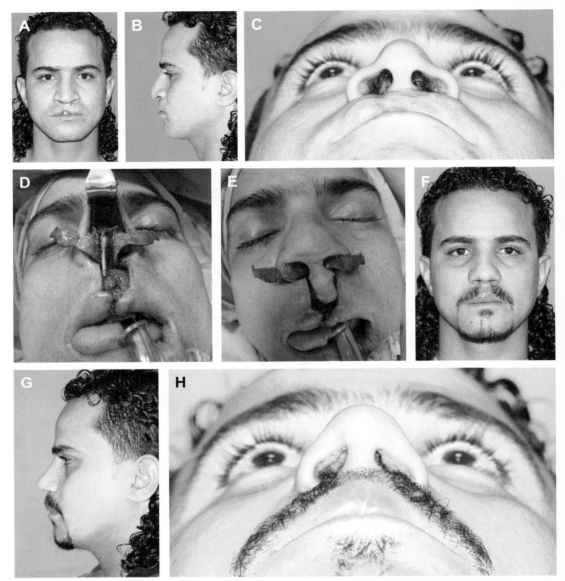

Fig. 2. Front, lateral, and base views (*A–C*) of a male patient with bilateral cleft lip nasal deformity demonstrating typical features of this type of nose dysmorphology. His rhinoplasty (*D–E*) was combined with lip redo. The prolabium was pedicled on the columella and raised as one unit on the terminal branch of anterior ethmoid arteries that were preserved in dissection during the open rhinoplasty approach. The alar cartilages were dissected off the underlying mucosa to reorient and steal from lateral crura to build up medial crura. Septal extension graft and tip structuring built the new nasal tip. Early postoperative front, lateral, and base views (*F–H*).

supporting bone on all aspects of the root surface when patients are orthodontically prepared for segmental advancement surgery.[18]

Alveolar bone grafting
Repair of the alveolar cleft begins in the mid to late mixed dentition before the eruption of missing canine and guided by the eruption of its counterpart in unilateral cases. It has been demonstrated in multiple studies to have no effect on midface growth.[19,20] ABG facilitates orthodontic space closure,[21] thus simplifying future orthognathic procedures. In a bilateral CL/P patient with a severely displaced premaxilla, surgical repositioning may be considered in conjunction with the ABG.[22,23]

Preorthognathic speech pathology assessment
The presurgical workup should include a speech pathology evaluation. This includes clinical evaluation as well as instrumental testing to assess the

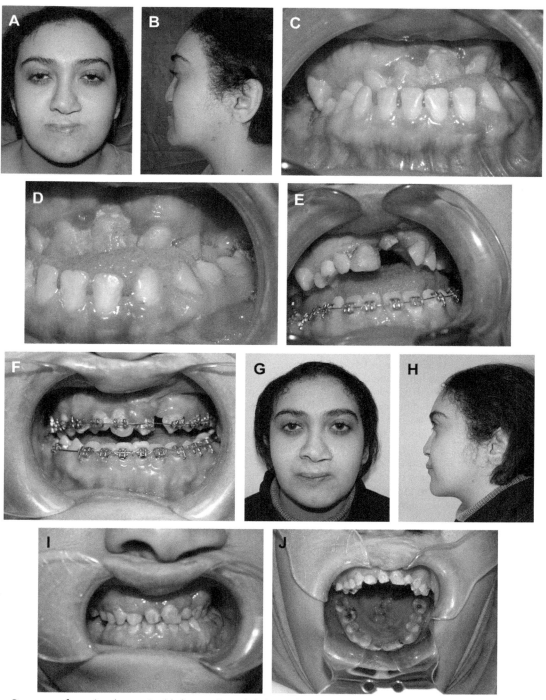

Fig. 3. a case of previously repaired left complete cleft lip and palate showing hypoplastic maxilla, a constricted maxillary dental arch, and class III malocclusion (A–D). Orthodontic preparation to expand the arch followed by alveolar bone grafting (E–G). Early postoperative front, lateral, and occlusion views following Le Fort I advancement (H–J).

risk of developing velopharyngeal insufficiency after surgery.[18]

Orthognathic Surgery

Surgical planning

Orthognathic surgery in the cleft patient mainly involves maxillary advancement with the possible mandibular setback. When indicated, bimaxillary surgery will reduce the magnitude of both the maxillary and the mandibular movements needed to correct the underlying skeletal imbalance.[3] This requires the fabrication of a surgical intermediate splint, for the relation of the new maxilla position to the existing mandible, and a final surgical splint, which relates the final mandibular position to the fixed final maxillary position.[24]

Virtual surgical planning

The ability to design osteotomies and advance skeletal elements freely and carry out unlimited trials of maneuvers in the preoperative simulated environment with precise anthropometrics of these manipulations has revolutionized the virtual surgical planning (VSP) phase of craniofacial reconstruction.[25] The full workflow for orthognathic surgery includes virtual planning of the surgical treatment, three-dimensional printing of customized surgical devices (surgical cutting guide and titanium fixation plates), and possible real-time intraoperative navigation.[26] A surgical cutting guide can be used during surgery to pilot the osteotomy line that had been planned preoperatively at the computer and the custom-made fixation titanium plates will allow the desired repositioning of the maxilla.[27]

Cleft orthognathic surgery has evolved from the simple maxillary Le Fort I advancement with the correction of dental malocclusion to the current model of patient-centered approach focusing on skeletofacial reconstruction using computer-assisted diagnosis and planning.[28] With the rising popularity of virtual surgical planning, there has been renewed interest in "mandible-first surgery" in certain circumstances including a cleft maxilla when double jaw surgery is indicated.[29,30] Three-dimensional imaging and surgical simulation have provided valuable information for facial aesthetics and surgical feasibility in the preoperative planning of complex cases. These include cases involving bimaxilla, multiple segments, multidirectional movements, or those involving distraction. When distraction has been planned, distraction devices can be carefully selected and modified. In this way, accurate planning of the distraction vector can be achieved.

Improved access and reduced costs have seen the use of virtual surgical planning expand,[3] and is, indeed, a tool to strive for perfection. VSP reduces the operation time, discomfort, and burden of care for patients and serves as an alternative to conventional model surgery in adult patients with CLP.[31] However, Wu and coworkers[32] reported outcome discrepancies from the virtual simulation of all rotational surgical corrections (roll, yaw, and pitch) being positively correlated to the degree of planned surgical movement and that patients with bilateral cleft lip and palate are more likely to incur outcome discrepancies in yaw correction with major maxillary advancement of more than 5 mm advancement. Similarly, Heifetz-Li and colleagues[33] documented a notable minority of points that were under-corrected in the anterior-posterior plane when using patient-specific osteotomy guides and plates, and recommended increased intraoperative clinical judgment when interpreting these deviations.

Le Fort I advancement (see Fig 3: g–j)

The Le Fort I osteotomy is performed in the standard fashion. A large amount of soft tissue scarring is common in cleft orthognathic patients. The most common symptom is a soft tissue constriction that restricts the mobility of the osteotomized maxilla. The application of constant and firm traction to the soft tissues limiting the maxillary advancement for a prolonged time is essential to achieve adequate advancement in many cleft cases.[3] In cases with more than 10 mm of advancement, soft tissue traction for 20 to 30 minutes may be required to ensure a passive seating of the maxilla into the interdental splint.[34] Mobilization and advancement are more difficult in bilateral CL/P cases. With large advancements, attention must be paid to the vascularity of the premaxilla. The mandibular teeth are wired into a prefabricated interdental splint, and the movable maxilla is subsequently inserted into the splint. Care must be given during this maneuver to ensure that the mandibular condyles are securely seated in the glenoid fossa. The maxilla is temporarily wired into the splint while the medial and lateral buttresses are rigidly fixed. The wires are removed and mouth opening is checked before closure.

Distraction osteogenesis

Maxillary distraction osteogenesis (DO) is now considered to be a valuable surgical option(Fig 4: e–i). In a recent study, the distraction group demonstrated greater maxillary advancement, less horizontal relapse of the maxilla, and higher life satisfaction when compared with the

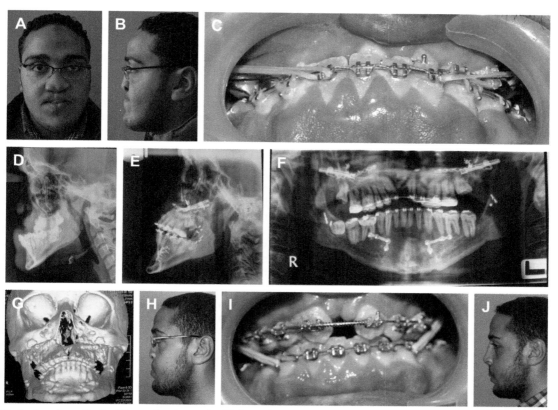

Fig. 4. A male patient with previously repaired bilateral complete cleft lip and palate who underwent double jaw orthognathic surgery elsewhere in his early teens with relapse and class III malocclusion (*A–D*). Readvancement of the maxilla was conducted using Le Fort I distraction (*E–G*). Lateral view (*H*) at the time of consolidation after reaching a functional occlusion (*I*). Six-months postoperative lateral views (*J*) following removal of distractors and augmentation rhinoplasty using rib graft and fat grafting of the upper lip to achieve facial balance.

osteotomy group.[35] Distraction osteogenesis would be indicated in a subset of cleft patients with severe maxillary deficit requiring anterior advancement of more than 10 mm. Nowadays, the technique of trans-sutural distraction osteogenesis (TSDO) is used to treat complex forms of craniofacial deformities and proved to be an effective tool for midface advancement, particularly in growing children with CLP.[36–38]

Postorthognathic Surgery

Postsurgical orthodontics
The occlusion is not required to be held in intermaxillary fixation (IMF) because skeletal stability following Le Fort I advancement is not dependent on postoperative IMF even in patients with CL/P.[39] Postoperative orthodontics is usually maintained for a period of 6 to 12 months.

Speech pathology follow-up
Postsurgical speech pathology assessment is indicated after removal of occlusal splint in the patient with an increased preoperative risk of velopharyngeal insufficiency.[3]

Complications
Relapse When compared with normal patient populations, the outcomes of well-coordinated orthognathic surgery for cleft patients can be excellent; nonetheless, there are greater risks of relapse(see **Fig 4**: a–d). Individuals with CL/P who received maxillary advancement by Le Fort I osteotomy and miniplate fixation had a 20% to 25% chance of relapse 1 year after surgery, compared with 10% in noncleft patients. This is due to scar tissue retraction, upper lip tightness, nasal septum interference, insufficient mobilization of the bony segment, and thin and fragile bony structures of the lateral pyriform wall and zygoma base for maintaining unyielding attachment.[34,40]

Velopharyngeal insufficiency It was reported that patients with normal speech have a 12.5% chance of developing velopharyngeal insufficiency after surgery. Hypernasality and borderline velopharyngeal insufficiency before surgery are risk factors for postoperative function impairment.[41,42]

Distraction osteogenesis Infection, malocclusion/relapse, avascular necrosis, and oronasal fistula recurrence are all complications related to distraction osteogenesis, similar to that in traditional orthognathic surgery. Device failure and skin irritation, on the other hand, are distractor-specific.[43]

Definitive Rhinoplasty

Definitive rhinoplasty is performed when all skeletal discrepancies have been addressed (**Fig. 1**: d–n and **2**: d–h). While an endonasal approach can bring improvements to cleft nose deformities, a successful outcome is more predictable when approached through an open technique.[11,38]

Incision
Trans-columellar open incision is the most common access technique in definitive rhinoplasty for cleft noses as it provides better exposure to the nasal lobule and septal cartilage as well as the underlying bony and soft tissue structures.[44] The traditional inverted-V incision can be modified to recruit upper lip skin to the columella with a V-to-Y closure or the incision can be made asymmetrically onto the nasal skin on the cleft side to recruit this skin inward to address a superomedial alar web.[38] To provide additional tissue to augment the vestibular lining and to diminish the alar-columellar web, a sliding chondrocutaneous flap allows tip stabilization and develops refinement.[45] A medial marginal columella incision is made approximately 1 to 2 mm from the columella edge and extends up to the domal recess. In the unilateral cleft, the rim incision is modified and placed closer to the skin margin.[11]

Septum
Correcting the septum involves resecting its cartilaginous and bony parts, including the vomer and perpendicular plate of the ethmoid bone.[11,46] In some cases, the septal deviation is too severe that the resection of the deviated segment and its replacement with a straight graft is necessary. The graft is obtained from the septal cartilage, or the rib cartilage may be used if a larger segment is needed.[15] Spreader grafts and batten onlay grafts may be harvested from the resected parts of the quadrangular septal cartilage, but most often are obtained from the curved portion of the right sixth rib to have an adequate shape, size, and strength of cartilage required in the cleft rhinoplasty.[47]

Spreader graft
Spreader grafts are placed between the septum and upper lateral cartilage bilaterally and fixated with sutures.[7,46] If required, the spreader graft can extend more caudally and act as a septal extension graft (SEG) for better nasal tip support as well as aiding in septum stability and straightening.

Nasal dorsum and nasal bone osteotomies
The nasal dorsum in cleft patients is often deficient and less pronounced when compared with non-cleft patients. Asymmetric osteotomies are used to correct the resultant bony pyramid deviation. Asymmetric osteotomies allow a wedge resection of the bony nasal pyramid to restore the difference between the long and short nasal sidewalls.[48] The nasal dorsal deficiency can also be addressed by using a dorsal onlay rib graft. Alternatively, silicone implants are used, but are not considered the standard of care in patients with CLP due to the higher incidence of postoperative complications.[49]

Lower lateral cartilage, batten grafts, and the nasal tip
The LLC collapses vertically and is positioned inferiorly in cleft nose deformities. A minimum of 5 to 7 mm of cartilage must be available for adequate tip support. Lateral crural steal (LCS) technique can be used in rhinoplasties of both unilateral and bilateral cleft lip and palate cases. The LCS is achieved by increasing the length of the medial crura by sacrificing the length of the lateral crura. The lateral crura are advanced medially in a curvilinear manner to allow the tip to be rotated superiorly and anteriorly, thus improving tip projection and symmetry.[49] To create an excellent nasal tip projection and definition, a shield graft and SEG can be applied. It is recommended that these grafts are harvested from either the septum or the rib cartilage because of the greater availability and quality of the cartilage as well as its ability to withstand postinflammatory changes.[50]

Pyriform rim and premaxilla augmentation
Rib graft, cortical bone graft, diced cartilage, silicone implant, or autologous fat grafting could be used to augment the appearance of the pyriform.[2,51]

Alar base
The alar base on the cleft side is displaced inferiorly and laterally. Various surgical techniques may be implemented to correct this displacement: V-Y advancement flap, sill resection, alar wedge resection (Weir procedure), and multiple suturing techniques.[38] A split-thickness skin graft or composite graft may be used in nostril enlargement to obtain symmetry.[49]

Autologous rib graft

For patients with cleft lip and palate, the autologous rib graft is the primary choice for the reconstruction of severe deformities, creation of nasal tip projection, and reinforcement of the underlying structures. The autologous rib graft is harvested from the right sixth or seventh rib; the left ribs are avoided because of proximity to the heart and the central portion of the rib is harvested to avoid warping.

Complications of cleft rhinoplasty

The intraoperative complications include bleeding and those related to anesthesia. Infection may occur as an early postoperative complication. Necrosis and wound dehiscence of the skin are extremely rare. Asymmetry is common, and patients should be informed that they might require additional surgery for further corrections. Granulomas, scar contracture, and synechia (both associated with nostril stenosis and nasal obstruction) are possible risks.[11] The most common late complication is persistent asymmetry at the level of nasal bones, nasal vault, tip of the nose, and, most commonly, at the alar base and nostril. The inability to produce sufficient nasal tip projection or loss of tip projection because of scarring is another common late complication resulting in supratip deformity and suboptimal tip definition. The main reason for this is postoperative tension within the tissue. Even a small amount of tension could drag the alar cartilage to its original position.[52] Other reported factors related to nose deformity recurrence are tissue scarring, memory of the alar cartilage, and differential growth between the cleft and noncleft sides.[39] Septal deviation can also recur, or there could be some residual (uncorrected) septal deviation caused by the magnitude of the primary deformity. Nevertheless, patients with cleft lip rhinoplasty benefit from surgery tremendously and are generally accepting of residual imperfections, especially if their breathing has improved.[7]

Adjuvant Therapies

The adjuvant therapies include the use of fillers and autologous fat allowing for the enhancement of a deficient lip or philtral ridge on the cleft side, thus vastly improving the overall outcome (see Fig 4: j). These procedures provide a synergistic overall improvement in the results with rhinoplasty for patients with cleft lip and palate.[39]

SUMMARY

Orthognathic surgery is one of the many treatment modalities to address the functional and cosmetic challenges of patients with cleft lip and palate. It necessitates careful planning that involves all members of the multidisciplinary care team. To correct the dentofacial and skeletal abnormalities associated with congenital clefting and resultant scarring, maxillary advancement with or without mandibular setback is often required. The maxillary advancement can be achieved through traditional Le Fort I osteotomy, or in severe cases, distraction osteogenesis could be performed. Rhinoplasties in cleft patients are usually performed after the skeletal discrepancies are corrected. Cleft rhinoplasty is one of the most challenging and arduous procedures among different rhinoplasties. However, it allows a remarkable improvement in the patients' symmetry, esthetics and enhances function, thus improving the holistic quality of life of cleft patients.

CLINICS CARE POINTS

- When evaluating a patient with cleft lip nose deformity for rhinoplasty, one must assess speech, evaluate for nasal airway, and examine the position of underlying maxilla.

- If the amount of maxillary advancement needed exceeds 10 mm, distraction osteogenesis (DO) or bimaxillary surgery can be considered depending on the analysis of underlying skeletal imbalance.

- If there is an adapted functional occlusion and minimal maxillary retrusion, one might consider pyriform rim and premaxilla augmentation over orthognathic osteotomies.

- When performing orthognathic surgery, mouth opening is checked before incision closure to ensure achieving the desired occlusion and secure mandibular condyles seating in the glenoid fossa.

- When using patient-specific osteotomy guides and plates, it is recommended to increase intraoperative clinical judgment when interpreting any deviations from the virtual plan.

- The open approach for definitive rhinoplasty has many advantages and the incision is modified to become closer to the margin of skin and designed to recruit additional tissue to help achieve lower nasal third symmetry.

- Cartilage is required in the cleft rhinoplasty, so always be prepared to harvest autogenous rib grafts. Using the central portion of the rib reduces the chances of warping.

- Consider asymmetric osteotomies to correct the bony pyramid deviation and dorsal onlay rib graft to address nasal dorsal deficiency.
- To better support nasal tip and straighten the septum, extend the spreader graft more caudally to serve as a septal extension graft (SEG).
- To improve tip projection and symmetry, consider using lateral crural steal technique and a shield graft.
- The adjuvant therapies as the use of fillers and autologous fat can improve the overall results.

DISCLOSURE

The authors have nothing to disclose.

REFERENCES

1. Olds CE, Sykes JM. Cleft Rhinoplasty. Clin Plast Surg 2022;49(1):123–36.
2. Kaufman Y, Buchanan EP, Wolfswinkel EM, et al. Cleft nasal deformity and rhinoplasty. Semin Plast Surg 2012;26(4):184–90.
3. Roy AA, Rtshiladze MA, Stevens K, et al. Orthognathic surgery for patients with cleft lip and palate. Clin Plast Surg 2019;46(2):157–71.
4. Bardach J, Cutting C. Anatomy of unilateral and bilateral cleft lip and nose. In: Bardach J, Morris HL, editors. Multidisciplinary management of cleft lip and palate. Philadelphia: Saunders; 1990. p. 154–8.
5. Haddock NT, McRae MH, Cutting CB. Long-term effect of primary cleft rhinoplasty on secondary cleft rhinoplasty in patients with unilateral cleft lip-cleft palate. Plast Reconstr Surg 2012;129:740–8.
6. Garfinkle JS, King TW, Grayson BH, et al. A 12-year anthropometric evaluation of the nose in bilateral cleft lip-cleft palate patients following nasoalveolar molding and cutting bilateral cleft lip and nose reconstruction. Plast Reconstr Surg 2011;127: 1659–67.
7. Allori AC, Mulliken JB. Evidence-based medicine: Secondary correction of cleft lip nasal deformity. Plast Reconstr Surg 2017;140:166e–76e.
8. Saleh MA, Elshahat A, Emara M, et al. Objective Tools to Analyze the Lower Lateral Cartilage in Unilateral Cleft Lip Nasal Deformities. J Craniofac Surg 2011;22(4):1435–9.
9. Allori AC, Marcus JR. Modern tenets for repair of bilateral cleft lip. Clin Plast Surg 2014;41:179–88.
10. Cuzalina A, Jung C. Rhinoplasty for the cleft lip and palate patient. Oral Maxillofac Surg North Am 2016; 28(2):189–202.
11. Guyuron B. M.O.C.-P.S.(S.M.) CME article: Late cleft lip nasal deformity. Plast Reconstr Surg 2008; 121(Suppl):1–11.
12. Yoshimura Y, Okumoto T, Iijima Y, et al. Reduced nasal growth after primary nasal repair combined with cleft lip surgery. J Plast Reconstr Aesthet Surg 2015;68:e159–66.
13. Susami T, Kuroda T, Amagasa T. Orthodontic treatment of a cleft palate patient with surgically assisted rapid maxillary expansion. Cleft Palate Craniofac J 1996;33(5):445.
14. Phillips JH, Klaiman P, Delorey R, et al. Predictors of velopharyngeal insufficiency in cleft palate orthognathic surgery. Plast Reconstr Surg 2005;115(3):681–6.
15. Brattstrom V, McWilliam J, Larson O, et al. Craniofacial development in children with unilateral clefts of the lip, alveolus, and palate treated according to four different regimes. I. Maxillary development. Scand J Plast Reconstr Surg Hand Surg 1991;25(3):259–67.
16. Good PM, Mulliken JB, Padwa BL. Frequency of Le-Fort I osteotomy after repaired cleft lip and palate of cleft palate. Cleft Palate Craniofac J 2007;44(4): 396–401.
17. Posnick JC, Tompson B. Modification of the maxillary Le Fort I osteotomy in cleft-orthognathic surgery: the bilateral cleft lip and palate deformity. J Oral Maxillofac Surg 1993;51(1):2–11.
18. Leshem D, Tompson B, Phillips JH. Segmental LeFort I surgery: turning a predicted soft-tissue failure into a success. Plast Reconstr Surg 2006;118(5):1213–6.
19. Semb G. Effect of alveolar bone grafting on maxillary growth in unilateral cleft lip and palate patients. Cleft Palate J 1988;25(3):288–95.
20. Daskalogiannakis J, Ross RB. Effect of alveolar bone grafting in the mixed dentition on maxillary growth in complete unilateral cleft lip and palate patients. Cleft Palate Craniofac J 1997;34(5):455.
21. Cassolato SF, Ross B, Daskalogiannakis J, et al. Treatment of dental anomalies in children with complete unilateral cleft lip and palate at SickKids hospital, Toronto. Cleft Palate Craniofac J 2009;46(2):166.
22. Aburezq H, Daskalogiannakis J, Forrest C. Management of the prominent premaxilla in bilateral cleft lip and palate. Cleft Palate Craniofac J 2006;43(1): 92–5.
23. Geraedts CT, Borstlap WA, Groenewoud JM, et al. Long-term evaluation of bilateral cleft lip and palate patients after early secondary closure and premaxilla repositioning. Int J Oral Maxillofac Surg 2007; 36(9):788–96.
24. Levy-Bercowski D, DeLeon E Jr, Stockstill JW, et al. Orthognathic cleft-surgical/orthodontic treatment. Semin Orthod 2011;17(3):197–206.
25. Kalmar KL, Xu W, Zimmerman CE, et al. Trends in Utilization of Virtual Surgical Planning in Pediatric Craniofacial Surgery. J Craniofac Surg 2020;31: 1900–5.

26. Lo L-J, Lin H-H. Three-dimensional computer-assisted surgical simulation and intraoperative navigation in orthognathic surgery: a literature review. J Formos Med Assoc 2015;114:300e–7e.

27. Mazzoni S, Bianchi A, Schiariti G, et al. Computer-aided design and computer-aided manufacturing cutting guides and customized titanium plates are useful in upper maxilla waferless repositioning. J Oral Maxillofac Surg 2015;73:701–7.

28. Denadai R, Pai BCJ, Lo L-J. Balancing the dental occlusion and facial aesthetic features in cleft orthognathic surgery: patientcentered concept for computer-aided planning. Biomed J 2020;43:143–5.

29. Borba AM, Borges AH, PS C, et al. Mandible-first sequence in bimaxillary orthognathic surgery: a systematic review. Int J Oral Maxillofac Surg 2016;45:472–5.

30. Naran S, Steinbacher DM, Taylor JA. Current concepts in orthognathic surgery. Plast Reconstr Surg 2018;141:925e.

31. Wang Y, Li J, Xu Y, et al. Accuracy of virtual surgical planning-assisted management for maxillary hypoplasia in adult patients with cleft lip and palate. JPRAS 2020;73:134–40.

32. Wu T-J, Lee Y-H, Chang Y-J, et al. Three-dimensional outcome assessments of cleft lip and palate patients undergoing advancement plast, 2019 maxillary advancement plast. Reconstr Surg 2019;143:1255e.

33. Heifetz-Li JJ, Mechas N, Deitrick P. How accurate are patient-specific osteotomy guides and fixation plates in orthognathic surgery? Adv Oral Maxillofac Surg 2021;3:100124.

34. Posnick JC, Dagys AP. Skeletal stability and relapse patterns after Le Fort I maxillary osteotomy fixed with miniplates: the unilateral cleft lip and palate deformity. Plast Reconstr Surg 1994;94(7):924–32.

35. Kloukos D, Fudalej P, Sequeira-Byron P, et al. Maxillary distraction osteogenesis versus orthognathic surgery for cleft lip and palate patients. Cochrane Database Syst Rev 2018;8:CD010403.

36. Tong H, Gao F, Yin J, et al. Three-dimensional quantitative evaluation of midfacial skeletal changes after trans-sutural distraction osteogenesis for midfacial hypoplasia in growing patients with cleft lip and palate. J Cranio Maxill Surg 2015;43:1749–57.

37. Liu C, Liu C, Gao Q, et al. Transsutural distraction osteogenesis versus osteotemy distraction osteogenesis. J Craniofac Surg 2012;23:464–71.

38. Sykes J, Senders C, Wang T, et al. Use of the open approach for repair of secondary cleft lip nasal deformity. Fac Plast Surg North Am 1993;1:111–26.

39. Lo LJ. Primary correction of the unilateral cleft lip nasal deformity: achieving the excellence. Chang Gung Med J 2006;29:262–7.

40. Welch TB. Stability in the correction of dentofacial deformities: a comprehensive review. J Oral Maxillofac Surg 1989;47(11):1142–9.

41. Janulewicz J, Costello BJ, Buckley MJ, et al. The effects of Le Fort I osteotomies on velopharyngeal and speech functions in cleft patients. J Oral Maxillofac Surg 2004;62(3):308–14.

42. Witzel MA, Munro IR. Velopharyngeal insufficiency after maxillary advancement. Cleft Palate J 1977;14(2):176–80.

43. Cheung LK, Chua HD. A meta-analysis of cleft maxillary osteotomy and distraction osteogenesis. Int J Oral Maxillofac Surg 2006;35(1):14–24.

44. Daskalogiannakis J, Mehta M. The need for orthognathic surgery in patients with repaired complete unilateral and complete bilateral cleft lip and palate. Cleft Palate Craniofac J 2009;46(5):498–502.

45. Wang TD, Madorsky SJ. Secondary rhinoplasty in nasal deformity associated with the unilateral cleft lip. Arch Facial Plast Surg 1999;1(1). https://doi.org/10.1001/archfaci.1.1.40.

46. Ross RB. Treatment variables affecting facial growth in complete unilateral cleft lip and palate. Cleft Palate J 1987;24(1):5–77.

47. Adlam DM, Yau CK, Banks P. A retrospective study of the stability of midface osteotomies in cleft lip and palate patients. Br J Oral Maxillofac Surg 1989;27(4):265–76.

48. Ince B, Dadaci M. Base nasal bone resection versus oblique nasal bone resection: a comparative study of the outcome for the deviated nose. Plast Reconstr Surg 2017;139:29e–37e.

49. Cuzalina A, Tolomeo PG. Challenging rhinoplasty for the cleft lip and palate patient. Oral Maxillofacial Surg Clin N Am 2021;33(1):143–59.

50. Cuzalina A, Tamim A. Cleft lip and palate patient rhinoplasty. In: Contemporary rhinoplasty. London, UK: IntechOpen; 2019.

51. Liang Y, Wang X. Application of diced autologous rib cartilage for paranasal augmentation in cleft nose. Aesth Plast Surg 2021;45(3):1169–75.

52. Huang H, Li Y, Cheng X, et al. Mechanical analysis of critical maneuvers in the correction of cleft lip nasal deformity. PLoS One 2018;13(4):e0195583.

Adjunctive Aesthetic Procedures in Orthognathic Surgery

Johan Jansma, MD, DDS, MSc, PhD, FEBOMFS[a,b,*],
Rutger H. Schepers, MD, DDS, MSc, PhD[a,b]

KEYWORDS

- Fat grafting • Liposuction • Blepharoplasty • Lip lift • Injectables • Facial implants • Aging
- Aesthetic

KEY POINTS

- To reach the best outcome of orthognathic surgery it is of importance to have knowledge not only of correct occlusion but also of facial balance, beauty, and harmony.
- To improve facial balance, harmony, and beauty, surgeons should have knowledge of adjunctive facial aesthetic procedures and their possible outcomes.
- The ability to combine aesthetic procedures with orthognathic planning and surgery may enhance patient satisfaction and will make one a more complete surgeon.

INTRODUCTION

Aesthetics play an important role in the planning and performance of orthognathic surgery, along with function, occlusion, and airway. An important aesthetic goal in orthognathic planning is to improve facial balance, harmony, volume, and symmetry. It is therefore logical that adjunctive aesthetic procedures become a part of the overall orthognathic treatment plan and that their possibilities are discussed with orthognathic candidates. There is no consensus on what facial beauty is because it differs with time, between cultures, and between people. Professionals like to develop and use all kinds of measurements and analyses to try to objectively determine facial beauty and facial harmony, and thereby to provide guidelines for the planning of orthognathic and other types of facial surgery (**Fig. 1**). Although there are different analyses at clinicians' disposal, it is preferred not to treat patients by numbers but rather try to help them become the most beautiful version of themselves. Despite the paradigm shift from two-dimensional orthognathic planning in profile view to more advanced three-dimensional (3D) virtual planning, clinical experience and artistry are still helpful in this respect.

Facial beauty and/or facial rejuvenation enhancement are the two most important reasons for opting for aesthetic facial surgery. These also apply to orthognathic surgery, along with functional improvement. The aim of many aesthetic procedures is to increase or change the volume in different regions of the face (eg, fat grafting, osteotomies of the malar region, alloplastic implants, liposuction), whereas for some it is to change the shape of certain facial parts (eg, rhinoplasty, otoplasty, lip fillers). Facial aging is a process that starts after the age of 25 and generally follows a standard pattern (**Fig. 2**). Individual variations and the severity of the aging process are not only influenced by genetic factors but also by environmental factors, such as smoking habits and sunlight exposure. There are roughly four factors

[a] Department of Oral and Maxillofacial Surgery, University Medical Center Groningen, PO Box 30.001, Groningen 9700RB, the Netherlands; [b] Department of Oral and Maxillofacial Suregry, Expert Center for Orthofacial Surgery, Martini Hospital Groningen, PO Box 30.033, Groningen, the Netherlands
* Corresponding author.
E-mail address: j.jansma@umcg.nl

Oral Maxillofacial Surg Clin N Am 35 (2023) 139–152
https://doi.org/10.1016/j.coms.2022.06.007
1042-3699/23/© 2022 Elsevier Inc. All rights reserved.

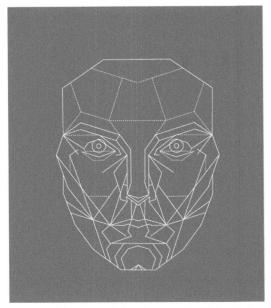

Fig. 1. Golden proportion face mask. This mask as developed by Dr Marquardt is based on the mathematical ratio of 1:1.618 (golden ratio) that appears recurrently in beautiful things in nature. The mask is an attempt to understand and quantify the perfect, ideal, or most beautiful facial proportions regardless of age or time.

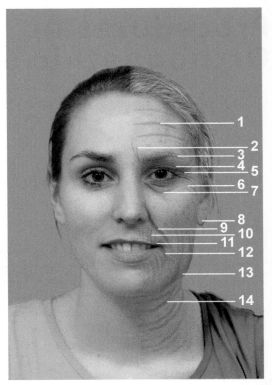

Fig. 2. Artist animation of facial aging. (1) Forehead wrinkles. (2) Frown lines. (3) Brow ptosis. (4) Dermatochalasis. (5) Lateral hooding. (6) Crow's feet. (7) Tear troughs. (8) Earlobe enlargement. (9) Deepening nasolabial folds. (10) Lengthening of upper lip. (11) Lip lines. (12) Marionette lines. (13) Jowling. (14) Neck wrinkles.

involved in facial aging: (1) loss of volume (deflation), (2) displacement of tissues, (3) loss of elasticity, and (4) skin changes. Orthognathic advancement surgery of either jaw increases the facial volume, thus having an antiaging effect on younger patients and a rejuvenating effect on older individuals. Advancement of the maxillomandibular complex can enhance lip support, reduce nasolabial folds, and reduce jowling. Bimaxillary advancement, with or without genioplasty, is therefore often referred to as a reversed facelift (**Fig. 3**). Some aesthetic volumizing procedures can help with enhancing the volume further in different aesthetic regions of the face (eg, by fat grafting and malar augmentation), whereas those procedures aimed at removing redundant tissue can also create a more youthful appearance (eg, lip lift, blepharoplasty, and liposuction).

Aesthetic procedures are categorized as: (1) procedures that enhance the results of orthognathic surgery, and can be performed concomitantly; (2) procedures performed secondarily after a soft tissue edema has resolved and healing is complete; (3) procedures that can address undesired aesthetic changes that have occurred after orthognathic surgery; and (4) procedures that are performed to camouflage certain aspects in patients not desiring optimal orthognathic surgery.[1]

In this article, we discuss different facial aesthetic procedures that are combined with orthognathic surgery, to the patient's benefit, to help them become the most beautiful version of themselves. This overview is not extensive because certain procedures are covered elsewhere in this issue.

FACIAL FAT GRAFTING

Autologous facial fat transplantation, a commonly applied procedure in aesthetic surgery since the 1980s, is an easy to use, effective, and safe technique with a low complication rate and minimal donor-site morbidity.[2] The latter is because subcutaneous fat is abundantly available in most patients, and is fully biocompatible and conceivably permanent. However, fat grafting studies have reported between 25% and 80% long-term volume retention. This variable amount of volume retention is one of the major disadvantages of the technique and often necessitates repeated surgical

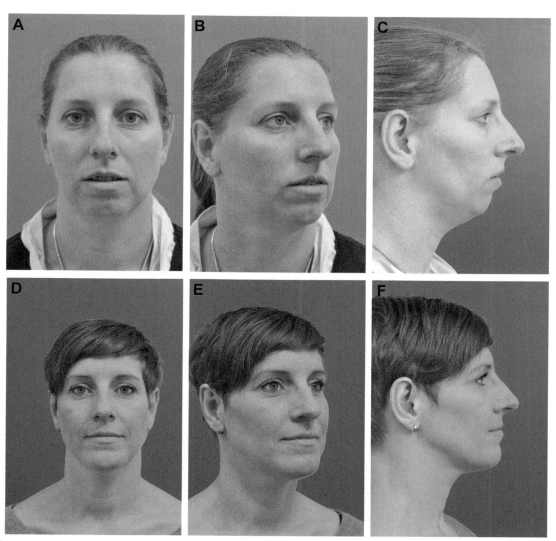

ig. 3. Female patient (36 years old) with mandibular retrognathia and obtuse cervical angle and nose-lip angle. he underwent combined orthodontic and surgical treatment consisting of bimaxillary advancement with coun- erclockwise rotation and advancement genioplasty. No adjunctive aesthetic procedure was performed. The or- ognathic surgery has led to an increased facial volume and improvement of the profile, sometimes referred to s reversed facelift. Preoperative situation in frontal (*A*), three-quarter (*B*), and profile view (*C*). Postoperative sit- ation in frontal (*D*), three-quarter (*E*), and profile view (*F*).

procedures, so called touch-up procedures.[3] Nevertheless, the volumizing effect of lipofilling is ubtle and soft, creating a more youthful appear- nce, especially in the periorbital and zygomatic rea (**Fig. 4**). Before starting the procedure, the pa- ent should be examined in an upright position nd markings should be made on the area of the kin with a volume deficit to accentuate the area f the planned correction. A series of preopera- vely made patient photographs should be avail- ble during the process to help in evaluating the lan and the progress of the correction. The

procedure starts with injecting the donor site with an infiltration solution (Ringer solution or sodium nitrate combined with lidocaine 2%) followed by gentle manual liposuction, usually using a 10-mL Luer lock syringe, 2-mL negative pressure, and a blunt cannula with a small diameter (2.4 mm) and small holes. The fat is then processed with centri- fugation, washing, or decantation techniques. Recent research points to a slightly beneficial outcome, regarding fat cell viability, from the washing method.[4] The fat is subsequently injected into the subcutaneous tissues of the target areas

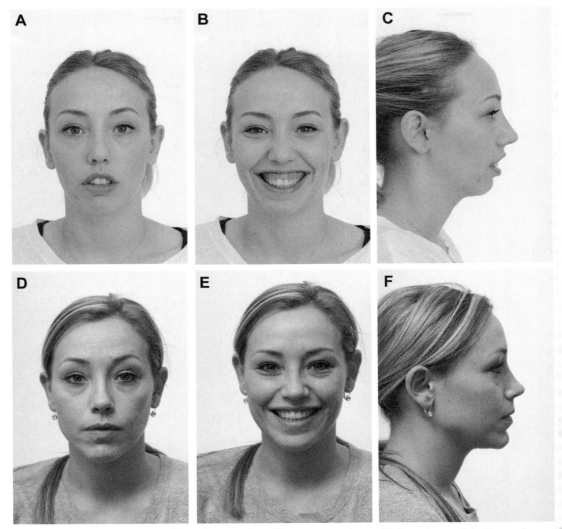

Fig. 4. Female patient (27 years old) with vertical maxillary excess and mandibular retrognathia. She underwent combined orthodontic and surgical treatment consisting of bimaxillary osteotomy with maxillary impaction, mandibular advancement, and advancement genioplasty. As an adjunctive procedure fat grafting (7 mL per side) of the zygoma and infraorbital regions was performed to enhance definition. Preoperative situation in frontal (*A, B*) and profile view (*C*). Postoperative situation in frontal (*D, E*) and profile view (*F*).

of the face using a small blunt cannula (0.9–1.2 mm diameter). According to a recent study, there is site-dependent variation in volumetric retention after facial fat grafting, with the zygoma area showing a 40% volumetric effect 1 year post-treatment compared with an unmeasurable volumetric effect in the lip area using a 3D measuring method.[3]

To enhance volume retention of the grafted fat, several fat enrichment strategies are being investigated, including adding: adipose tissue–derived stromal cells; tissue stromal vascular fraction; cellular stromal vascular fraction; and nanofat, microfat, and platelet-rich plasma or fibrin to the grafted fat. Even though some studies show a promising beneficial effect of these additives regarding volume retention, high-quality research, with proper volumetric measurements, is lacking. Fat grafting results in excellent soft volume enhancement, which is beautiful.[2] However, fat grafting does not always provide enough projection, for instance to enhance the cheekbone area. In such situations, the fat can be too soft in its augmenting effect. Facial implants, or an intraoral zygoma osteotomy, can then be indicated. Fat grafting can also be used as an adjunctive procedure to implant placement or zygoma osteotomy to create more projection and softness. When combined with an osteotomy, the fat grafting procedure should, preferably, be performed immediately after the osteotomy so the apparent effect of the osteotomy on the face can then be taken into account and swelling has not yet occurred.

SOFT TISSUE FILLERS

The use of soft tissue fillers has increased tremendously. In 2019, almost three-quarters of a million procedures were performed in the United States alone.[5] Soft tissue fillers are predominantly resorbable and basically have two variations: hyaluronic acid (HA) fillers and biostimulatory fillers. Since the Food and Drug Administration approved Restylane (Q-med, Uppsala, Sweden) as an HA filler in 2003, most of the currently used fillers consist of HAs. HA fillers are based on glycosaminoglycan chains that coil in on themselves, resulting in a viscous and elastic matrix that is hydrophilic in nature. These fillers are easy to apply, not time consuming, and inexpensive. HA fillers also have an overall low rate of adverse events.[6] The filler degrades over time, with the amount of cross-linking between the glycosaminoglycan chains theoretically changing the clinical half-life. Hence, the volumetric effect of HA fillers varies from 1 to 3 years, depending on the amount of cross-linking and other aspects of the filler, with the maximum effect occurring 1 to 3 months post-treatment. Soft tissue fillers are, in general, applied under local anesthesia in a precise manner using a needle or a cannula varying from 23 to 30 gauge. In the beginning, fillers were predominantly used to smooth out wrinkles but, over the last decade they have evolved into contour and shape defining fillers. The disadvantage of HA fillers, compared with fat grafting, is that the volumetric effect is not permanent, even though some authors claim a collagen stimulatory effect. The advantage over fat grafting is the constant and predictable volumetric effect, which is fairly equivalent in all the soft tissue layers. Therefore, HA fillers are indicated more for the lips than fat grafting (**Fig. 5**) and may be more effective for subtle defects, such as an A-frame deformity of the upper eyelid, marionette lines, prejowl depression, and mental creases. However, a too superficial injection, such as under the thin skin of the lower eyelid, can cause a blue discoloration of the skin called Tyndall effect, which is thought to occur because of stronger scattering of the blue light spectrum through the colloid particles.

Even though the volumizing effect of some HA fillers lasts for several years, it usually decreases over time, necessitating, as sometimes with fat grafting, touch-up treatments to maintain the desired result. HA filler treatment can be done immediately following an osteotomy, but it is generally performed postoperatively because the procedure is tolerated well and usually smaller volumes are applied compared with lipofilling. Therefore, applying the HA filler 3 to 6 months postoperatively when the edema has largely resolved, and the result of the osteotomy is examined while the patient is in an upright position, is usually preferred. It can even be beneficial to wait with lip augmentation until the orthodontic procedure has been completed and the orthodontic appliances taken out to rule out any projection caused by the appliance on the lips. Application of a lip filler can also compensate for the lack of dental lip support. Small imperfections that remain after, or are caused by the orthognathic surgery, can also be corrected in this manner.[7]

FACIAL IMPLANTS

Alloplastic facial implants are easily combined with orthognathic surgery, especially because most implants can be placed subperiosteally through the intraoral incisions that are being used for the orthognathic procedure. Implants can correct bony deficits in a rigid manner, giving a firm projection that mimics the projection of bone and simulates a bony feeling when palpated. Off-the-shelf facial implants are available in different shapes and sizes corresponding to various areas of the face lacking projection. They are modified, if needed, in the operating room using a scalpel. Mandibular angle, chin, and zygoma are especially popular regions to augment. Facial implants are often made of solid silicone rubber, porous polyethylene, titanium, or polyether ether ketone (PEEK).[8] These implants, preferably fixated with screws, have stood the test of time and have proven to be safe. Complications are rare, mainly caused by bacterial biofilm formation and infection, usually leading to removal of the implant. Also, implant displacement can occur and, in time, resorption of the bone underlying the implant may result in loss of projection. Sterilizable 3D-printed bony models of the patient are helpful intraoperatively to estimate how and where the implant has to be modified. This is hard to judge in the patient during the surgery. The evolution of 3D planning has also led to more attention to patient-specific implants (PSIs). PSIs are made from several materials but are mostly made from polyether ether ketone. When combined with 3D

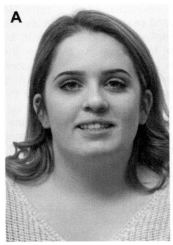
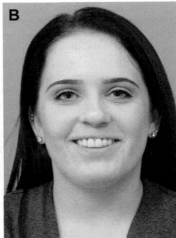
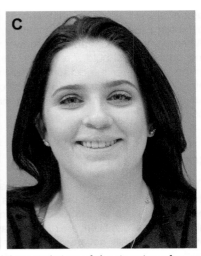

Fig. 5. Female patient (20 years old) with bilateral cleft lip and palate. (*A*) Frontal view of the situation after orthodontic treatment without orthognathic surgery. (*B*) Frontal view of the situation after aesthetic dentistry with eight porcelain facings of the upper teeth and first premolars. (*C*) Situation 1 year after injection of 2 mL hyaluronic acid filler (Voluma, Juvederm, Allergan Inc, Irvine, CA) for improved upper lip projection and volumization. (*Courtesy of* Marco Gresnigt, DDS, PhD, Groningen, NL (Figure 5B))

osteotomy planning, PSIs give excellent opportunities to correct, for instance, bony asymmetries and shapes in individuals in a precise way. Despite orthognathic surgery being well planned and executed, and correcting asymmetries to a large extent, some asymmetries can remain, especially in the mandible because it is not symmetric. It has proven to be helpful to correct the remaining asymmetries by placing a PSI of the mandibular angle and inferior border. Such implants are fabricated based on mirroring the image of a computed tomography scan that is made around 6 months after the orthognathic procedure (**Fig. 6**). Nevertheless, soft tissue asymmetries are hard to correct fully with implants and one should consider addressing them with additional fat grafting or filler injections either during implant placement or at a later stage.

There are various reasons why facial implants are not used extensively in orthognathic patients, even though they can lead to improved results. First of all, orthognathic surgery is mostly performed in young adolescents with favorable soft tissue volumes. Osteotomies of the chin- and zygoma are usually effective in facilitating the needed correction in these patients. This is, of course, not the case for patients with congenital disorders or needing improvements in mandibular angle definition because this can only be done with angle implants. In older patients, volume loss, deflation and projection are corrected using implants that give more support in the deflated area (eg, chin implants with a prejowl extension and submalar/

zygoma implants). One has to realize that a bony osteotomy performed at a younger age is beautiful during the first few decades, but can become unfavorable as the patient ages because of a certain loss of soft tissue volume and elasticity. This is obvious for large maxillary impactions, leading to invisibility of the upper teeth, and for mandibular setbacks in people with poor chin-neck definitions, leading to submandibular excess. One should also realize that large chin advancements may help to create a prejowl depression once jowling starts at a later age. Because many maxillofacial surgeons are mainly acting as bone surgeons, they feel more comfortable with performing osteotomies than applying an implant. This is also probably influenced by the bad reputation that implants still seem to have, although not in our and many other surgeons' experience.

SUBMENTAL LIPOSUCTION/LIPECTOMY

Accumulation of submental fat can cause effacement of the cervicomental angle, which becomes even more profoundly visible in mandibular retrognathia cases. Performing an advancement of the mandible and/or a genioplasty can improve the cervicomental angle quite well. Reducing any palpable subcutaneous fat in the submental area can contribute to the result.[9] This can usually be achieved easily after orthognathic surgery using a liposuction cannula of approximately 15 cm in length and a diameter of approximately 3 mm, and preferably only a few suction holes near the

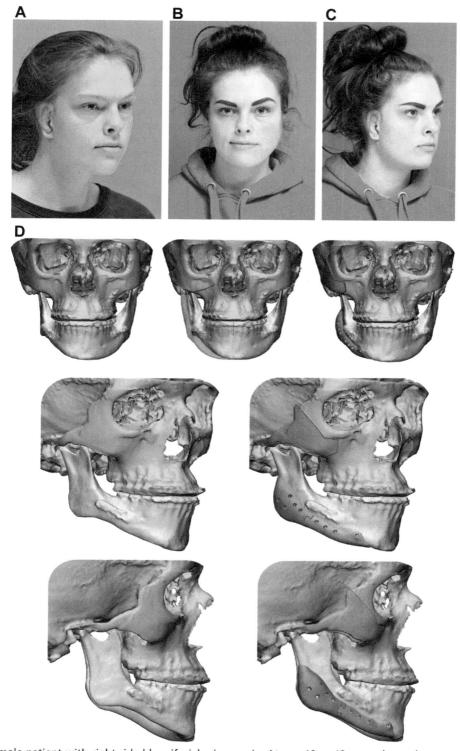

Fig. 6. Female patient with right-sided hemifacial microsomia. At age 10 to 12 years she underwent ear reconstruction elsewhere. At age 18 she underwent mandibular orthognathic surgery to correct the occlusion. At age 19 a PSI from polyether ether ketone was placed to increase the projection of the right mandibular angle and inferior border. This was combined with an intraoral zygoma osteotomy with outward rotation and fat

tip. A simple method to create the needed negative pressure of 30 to 50 mL is to use a Luer lock syringe. During the liposuction procedure, the plunger is locked using a simple clasp. Usually, 5 to 10 mL of fat is extracted via a small stab incision just behind the submental crease in the facial midline. One must keep in mind that the position of the hyoid plays an important role in the cervicomental angle. The lower and more anterior the hyoid bone is situated, the less one can expect from the visible effect of a submental liposuction on this angle. Besides this, the presence of platysma banding and skin laxity can also affect the outcome of the liposuction in a negative way. A lipectomy might be more effective for such cases or for when there is abundant submental fat extending to the anterior neck. This is performed through a small 2- to 3-cm incision just posterior of the submental crease, which also gives the opportunity to perform a corset platysmaplasty and anterior neck lift. All the mentioned submental procedures can be done under local anesthesia, but it is mostly beneficial to perform them following the orthognathic surgery while the patient is still under general anesthesia. Nevertheless, it is advocated to perform local anesthesia in the area to be treated because of the vasoconstrictive effect, thus minimizing the chance of a hematoma. Complications are rare because the critical structures are all underneath the platysma or deeper in the neck, except for the marginal branch of the facial nerve, which is at risk when penetrating the platysma. Postoperatively, great care should be taken to support the submental skin with an elastic bandage for a few days to prevent blood accumulation and sagging of the skin, both of which negatively influence the end result (**Fig. 7**).

OTOPLASTY

Misshapen and protruding ears may also bother patients who are in for orthognathic surgery. In most instances, the protrusion is caused by a combination of hyperplasia of the posterior conchal wall and lack of antihelical fold, with the latter playing a bigger role because of the antihelix not developing. To evaluate this, the ear has to be examined in different directions (front, behind, and side) and, preferably, measured. Behind the ear, from the mastoid area to the outer helical rim,

the superior aspect should measure 10 mm, and the middle portion (superior to the lobule) should measure 20 mm. Ears can be corrected as of 5 or 6 years of age and at any age in adulthood.

An ear correction begins at the posterior auricular crease. If an excision of the conchal bowl is also planned, the skin should be excised in an elliptical shape.[10] Although different procedures have been described, we prefer the Mustardé technique for creating the antihelical fold.[11] The Mustardé technique is done with or without scoring the scaphoid cartilage on the anterior auricle from the posterior approach. The antihelical fold is created using slowly resorbable matrass sutures equidistant and perpendicular to the planned fold position. The conchal bowl is resectioned in a kidney bean shaped fashion. Connective tissue and muscle attachments are removed down to the mastoid fascia so that the ear can be adapted to the cranial base passively using nonresorbable sutures. Our patients wear a compressive head wrap for 2 days after which they are instructed to wear a head band over the ears while sleeping for 2 additional weeks.

When combining otoplasty with orthognathic surgery, we prefer to perform the osteotomies first and then redrape for the ear surgery. The advantage of combining the procedures is that the healing and downtime are combined without compromising the results (**Fig. 8**).

BLEPHAROPLASTY

When looking at a face, the eyes are the first and most looked at feature. Eye-tracking studies confirm this; age judgements are made on preferential attention toward the eye region. The definition of a beautiful eye varies, but it is generally agreed that youthfulness correlates with attractiveness.[12] An eye is considered to be attractive when it has typical youthful features instead of aging ones. A beautiful, youthful eye is described as full and convex. Conversely, an aging eye appears hollower, because of volume loss and fat atrophy.

Eye region aesthetic surgery is therefore one of the most effective interventions to enhance facial aesthetics, with blepharoplasty of the upper eyelids being one of the most commonly performed procedures. The aim when doing the procedure

grafting of the infraorbital, zygomatic, and mandibular angle region (15 mL) on the right side. Situation before placement of the PSI in three-quarter (*A*) view. Situation (at age 23) after placement of the PSI, zygoma osteotomy, and fat grafting in frontal (*B*) and three-quarter (*C*) view. (*D*) From left to right, in frontal, three-quarter, and profile view the design of the polyether ether ketone implant consisting of two parts and the planning of the zygoma osteotomy is depicted.

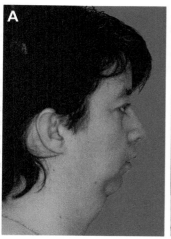
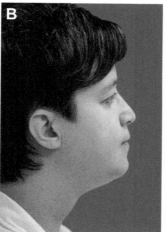
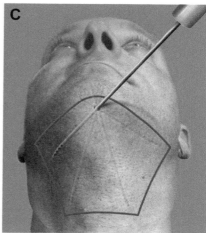

Fig. 7. Female patient (34 years old) with severe obstructive sleep apnea and mandibular retrognathia with obtuse cervical angle and fat deposition. She underwent combined orthodontic and surgical treatment consisting of counterclockwise bimaxillary advancement and advancement genioplasty. As an adjunctive procedure cervicofacial liposuction was performed to increase chin definition and improve the effect on the obstructive sleep apnea. (A) Profile view of the situation before combined treatment. (B) Profile view of the situation after orthognathic surgery and liposuction. Note the profile change. (C) Schematic drawing of the liposuction area bounded by the inferior mandibular border, the sternocleidoid muscles, and the hyoid.

on most aging patients is to correct skin excess (dermatochalasis) and lateral hooding.

In the past, surgeons were inclined to perform more invasive blepharoplasties, where excess skin was removed together with a strip of orbicularis oculi muscle, sometimes combined with excision or redistribution of fat from the medial and central fat compartments. Nowadays, surgeons tend to be more conservative and less invasive, by sparing the orbicularis oculi muscle and the orbital fat, because this preserves the fullness of the periorbital region, thus preventing the aged hollow orbit appearance.[13] Most of the patients just need the so-called skin-only procedure.

The preferred shape of the skin excision is not standard and varies from elliptical, lenticular S-shaped, and trapezoid to excisions that extend beyond the lateral orbital rim. Each surgeon has his/her own preference, and there is no consensus as to which is the most suitable blepharoplasty procedure, and for which patient.

The eyebrows are also an important part of the periorbital esthetic unit. In the diagnostic phase, it is important to determine their position and shape. Sometimes a browlift may be a better choice of treatment.[14]

Most orthognathic candidates are rather young and do not show signs of aging, whereas those older than the age of 40 can show signs of aging, and so an upper blepharoplasty may be indicated for them. The procedure is combined well with the osteotomy and takes about an extra 30 minutes.

We prefer to do the eyelid surgery after the osteotomy. The best results are attained by placing the markings for the upper eyelid incisions while the patient is in an upright position. This should be taken into account when combining the procedures. Care should also be taken when disinfecting and draping for the osteotomy so that the markings remain intact for the blepharoplasty. When performing a blepharoplasty under general anesthesia, local infiltration anesthesia is still warranted. This is also the case for cooling the eyelids during the first postoperative hours (**Fig. 9**).

LIP LIFT

The inclination of the upper teeth and orthognathic positioning of the maxilla influence lip position, lip shape, and tooth display, and should be considered when planning a combined treatment. A lip lift offers the possibility to rejuvenate the upper lip and to improve lip accent and appearance by eversion of the vermillion display.[15] The small single procedure can result in a large and noticeable change in the face, including a younger and more sensual appearance by shortening the perceived height of the midface, and by increasing the dental show of the upper arch. Most of the patients' nasolabial folds appear softer and shortened. Indications for the procedure include: a long or heavy upper lip; poor dental show; poor filler results (overfilled lips); filler complications; postsurgical drooping after rhinoplasty or orthognathic surgery;

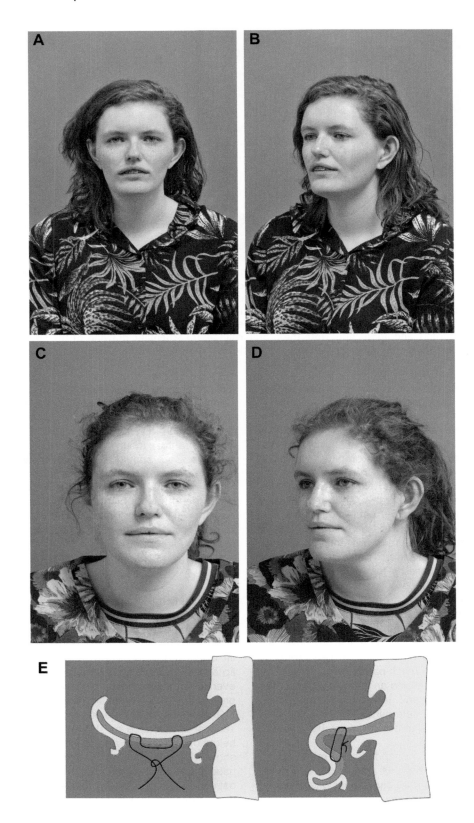

poorly defined or thin upper lip; mild asymmetry, especially of the Cupid's bow; and buried or drooping mouth corners. The patients often present with excessively long and drooping lips, looking tired and aged. An elongated upper lip can lengthen the appearance of the entire midface and, the longer the lip, the more likelihood of displaying diminished function while losing character and definition of the Cupid's bow. When planning the orthognathic surgery, it is often better to shorten a long upper lip rather than let it determine the position of the maxilla and upper teeth.

The so-called buffalo horn excision subnasal lip lift has already been in use for more than four decades, with a variety of personal modifications. Nasal base widening and atrophic scarring, striations and hypopigmentation are the most encountered postoperative problems. They seem to be mainly because of skin closure under tension and incision length and shape. It is therefore advocated by some authors to go for a deeper subsuperficial musculoaponeurotic system release and suspension of the superficial musculoaponeurotic system to the pyriform ligament to attain tension-free skin closure.[15]

While planning the lip lift, one should consider the overall facial balance by comparing the soft tissue proportions, and dental or skeletal predominance. A primary goal of the lip lift for most patients and surgeons is to increase the tooth show at rest and at function. Although a lack of tooth show exaggerates the aged appearance and can diminish sensuality, there is a turning point that must be respected for each patient, where the sensuality and youthfulness gained from an increase in tooth show and lip shortening transitions to a toothy or skeletonized appearance after excessive excision. There are no measurements or strict guidelines that would indicate this specific point. Rather than measuring the proportions directly, it is recommended to look at the face as a whole and simply envision the consequent changes. The overall intent is to make an appropriate lip fit in relation to its surrounding structures, especially the nose, cheeks, and chin.

Drawing the incision lines and determining the amount and shape of the skin excision are of paramount importance. The upper incision usually runs across the entire nasal base in the natural alar-facial and alar-labial crease. The incision continues under the nose, making sure not to invade the nasal sill. As a security measure, one can mark the minimum amount of remaining upper lip. This would, for most patients, be around 12 mm, measured from the Cupid's bow peak superiorly to the lower skin marking while the lip is on stretch mode. The amount to be excised ranges between 4 and 10 mm, with most excisions ranging between 5 and 7 mm. Excisions aiming for notable tooth show are typically between 7 and 9 mm. An excision of more than 10 mm is not advised because this dramatically increases healing time and makes redistribution of the skin difficult in the average patient. If there is a minor Cupid's bow asymmetry, it is corrected at this stage with an asymmetric excision. Lateral asymmetries cannot be corrected with a surgery centered at the base of the nose.[15]

The procedure can also be used for patients with adequate tooth show but who wish to improve their upper lip height, character, and volume. Even the most conservative lip lift can change the slope and vector of the vermillion, making it look like a lip filler has been applied.

A lip lift can be combined with some orthognathic surgeries (**Fig. 10**), including mandibular surgery if no other procedure is involved. The presence of a nasal tube is, however, a disadvantage so switching to an oral tube after the orthognathic procedure is considered. A lip lift should not be performed at the same time as a maxillary orthognathic procedure. Not only will the intraoral approach to the maxilla, and probably the swelling, have an influence, but also the healing process after repositioning the maxilla is somewhat unpredictable. Hence it is better to postpone the lip lift for those cases. We prefer to perform the lip lift as an outpatient procedure under local anesthesia once the brackets have been removed so that they do not influence the lip projection, and once the maxillary healing is complete (6 months at least).

Fig. 8. Female patient (24 years old) with mandibular retrognathia and a deep bite. She underwent combined orthodontic and surgical treatment consisting of clockwise bimaxillary advancement. As an adjunctive procedure the protruded left ear was corrected using Mustardé transcartilaginous nonresorbable sutures to increase the antihelical fold. Frontal (*A*) and three-quarter view with left ear (*B*) of the situation before surgery. Frontal (*C*) and three-quarter view from left side (*D*) after surgery and postoperative orthodontic treatment. (*E*) Schematic drawing of the Mustardé procedure with accentuation of the antihelical fold using transcartilaginous sutures from a posterior access.

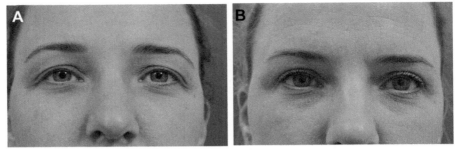

Fig. 9. Female patient (38 years old) with mild dermatochalasis of the upper eyelids (*A*). She underwent a skin-only upper blepharoplasty to improve the eyelid crease and to slightly increase the tarsal platform show. Note the subtle rejuvenating effect of the procedure (*B*).

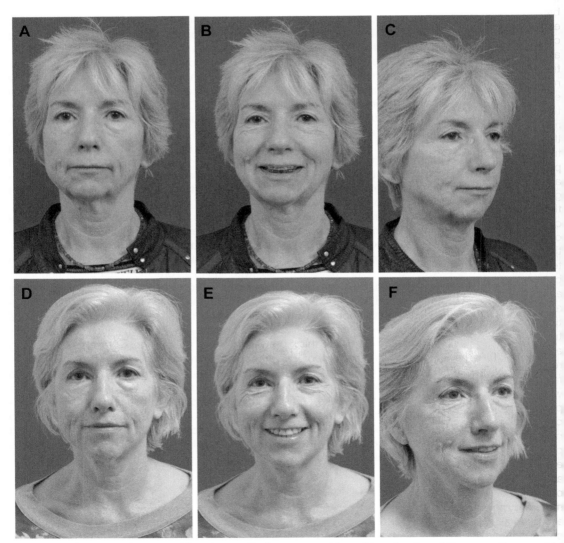

Fig. 10. Female patient (60 years old) with mandibular retrognathia and lengthening of the upper lip caused by facial aging. She underwent a combined orthodontic surgical treatment with mandibular advancement. The surgery was combined with a subnasal lip lift to shorten the upper lip and to evert the vermillion. Preoperative situation in frontal (*A*, *B*) and three-quarter view (*C*). Postoperative situation in frontal (*D*, *E*) and three-quarter view (*F*).

SUMMARY/DISCUSSION

Orthognathic surgery is much more than the correction of a malocclusion. The facial aesthetics also play an important role in patient satisfaction with the orthognathic surgery. Therefore, considerations regarding aesthetic factors should be discussed thoroughly with the patient and taken into account in every preoperative consultation and treatment planning. Even state-of-the-art planned and executed orthognathic procedures have their boundaries and shortcomings, and noticeable unfavorable side effects, such as mandible border irregularities and projection deficits. Discussing these possible outcome aspects with the patient beforehand not only prevents postoperative excuse conversations, but also highlights the great care taken by the surgeon in the process of achieving the best possible end result for the patient. Furthermore, this opens the door for mentioning additional esthetic procedures to either prevent unwanted outcomes or to improve treatment outcomes with respect to facial harmony, balance, and aesthetics, without making the patient feel that the surgeon is trying to sell extra procedures. Starting a discussion about the patient's facial aesthetics, and the possibility of adjunctive procedures, may be new to many surgeons because most of us are trained to base the discussion and treatment suggestions on the care demand expressed by the patient. In fact, in our experience, if one discusses aesthetics and the possibilities in a professional way, the patients tend to appreciate it. Nevertheless, one may be balancing on a thin line in that ethical issues may arise because, as a facial surgeon, one is biased and may foresee more small flaws in the outcome than the patient. One has to consider that under-treatment and overtreatment can result in unfavorable outcomes and/or unhappy patients. In this respect, care must be taken not to change the facial aspects of a patient in an overextensive way because it may even result in psychological problems for the patient in adapting to the facial changes. Thus, one has to keep this issue in mind when discussing the treatment options and planning before the orthognathic surgery in general, but maybe even more before performing adjunctive aesthetic procedures (especially in one procedure), because they can add up to a more profound outcome. Most adjunctive aesthetic procedures can, and are preferably, combined with the orthognathic surgery, especially when the outcome is expected to be good. From a practical point of view, this is beneficial for the patient. When in doubt whether to advocate an adjunctive aesthetic procedure or whether it is desired, it is much safer to refrain from doing it during the primary orthognathic surgery and plan it as a second-stage procedure after evaluating the outcome together with the patient. Besides clinical experience, 3D imaging and virtual surgical planning are a great help, especially for asymmetrical patients, despite that a lot of work still needs to be done regarding the accuracy of the soft tissue outcome predictabilities of the 3D surgical planning software. The 3D planning of adjunctive procedures, such as facial implant placement or fat grafting, is impossible in the currently available orthognathic virtual planning software. Despite the availability of planning software and all kinds of facial analyses, one would rather not treat by numbers and deliver unit sausage faces but rather help people become the best versions of themselves.

As with any type of nonsurgical or surgical procedure, training and experience are of utmost importance when offering and performing aesthetic facial surgery. Standard photo documentation of preoperative and postoperative situations is also of great importance when changing a patient's face.

In our view and experience, adjunctive aesthetic procedures to orthognathic surgery are beneficial for achieving great patient satisfaction. We believe that implementing these in an orthognathic practice helps in being more perceptive of all one's orthognathic patients' aesthetic aspects and the postoperative results. Finally, they lead to even more personal fulfilment after performing the orthognathic surgery.

CLINICS CARE POINTS

- There are roughly four factors involved in facial aging: loss of volume (deflation), displacement of tissues, loss of elasticity, and skin changes. Orthognathic advancement surgery of either jaw increases the facial volume, thus having an antiaging effect on younger patients and a rejuvenating effect on older individuals.

- Fat grafting studies have reported between 25% and 80% long-term volume retention. This variable amount of volume retention is one of the major disadvantages of the technique and often necessitates repeated surgical procedures, so called touch-up procedures.

- To enhance volume retention of the grafted fat, several fat-enrichment strategies are being investigated, including adding: adipose tissue derived stromal cells; tissue stromal vascular fraction; cellular stromal vascular fraction; and nanofat, microfat, and platelet-rich plasma or fibrin to the grafted fat. Even though some studies show a promising beneficial effect of these additives regarding volume retention, high-quality research, with proper volumetric measurements, is lacking.

- The advantage of hyaluronic acid (HA) fillers over fat grafting is the constant and predictable volumetric effect, which is fairly equivalent in all the soft tissue layers. Therefore, HA fillers are indicated more for the lips than fat grafting and may be more effective for subtle defects, such as an A-frame deformity of the upper eyelid, marionette lines, prejowl depression, and mental creases.

- A bony osteotomy performed at a younger age is beautiful during the first few decades, but can become unfavorable as the patient ages because of a certain loss of soft tissue volume and elasticity. This is obvious for large maxillary impactions, leading to invisibility of the upper teeth, and for mandibular setbacks in people with poor chin-neck definitions, leading to submandibular excess. Large chin advancements may help to create a prejowl depression once jowling starts at a later age.

- When looking at a face, the eyes are the first and most looked at feature. Eye-tracking studies confirm this; age judgements are made on preferential attention toward the eye region. Eye region aesthetic surgery is therefore one of the most effective interventions to enhance facial aesthetics, with blepharoplasty of the upper eyelids being one of the most commonly performed procedures.

- Care must be taken not to change the facial aspects of a patient in an overextensive way because it may even result in psychological problems for the patient in adapting to the facial changes.

- When in doubt whether to advocate an adjunctive aesthetic procedure or whether it is desired, it is much safer to refrain from doing it during the primary orthognathic surgery and plan it as a second-stage procedure after evaluating the outcome together with the patient.

DISCLOSURE

None of the authors has any commercial or financial conflicts of interest and has no funding sources.

REFERENCES

1. Mohamed WV, Perenack JD. Aesthetic adjuncts with orthognathic surgery. In: Spagnoli DB, Farrell BB, Tucker MR, editors. Orthognathic surgery. Oral and maxillofacial surgery clinics of north America. Philadelphia (PA): Elsevier; 2014. p. 573–85.
2. Coleman SR. Structural fat grafting. St. Louis (MO): Quality Medical Publishing; 2004.
3. Tuin AJ, Meulstee J, Loonen TGJ, et al. Three-dimensional facial volume analysis using algorithm-based personalized aesthetic templates. Int J Oral Maxillofac Surg 2020;49:1379–84.
4. Tuin AJ, Domerchie PN, Schepers RH, et al. What is the current optimal fat grafting processing technique? A systematic review. J Craniomaxillofac Surg 2016;44(1):45–55.
5. American Society for Aesthetic Plastic Surgery. Cosmetic surgery national data bank statistics 2019. Available at: https://www.surgery.org/sites/default/files/Aesthetic-Society_Stats2019Book_FINAL.pdf. Accessed October 25, 2020.
6. Stefura T, Kacprzyk A, Dros J, et al. Tissue fillers for the nasolabial fold area: a systematic review and meta-analysis of randomized clinical trials. Aesthetic Plast Surg 2021;45(5):2300–16.
7. Altamiro F. Dermal fillers for facial harmony. Batavia (IL): Quintessence Publishing; 2019.
8. Yaremchuk MJ, Chang CS, Dayan E, et al, editors. Atlas of facial implants. New York: Elsevier Inc; 2020.
9. Perez P, Hohman MH. Neck rejuvenation. In: StatPearls [Internet]. Treasure Island (FL): StatPearls Publishing; 2022.
10. Griffin JE, King K. Otoplasty. In: Griffin JE, King K, editors. Cosmetic surgery for the oral and maxillofacial surgeon. Chicago (IL): Quintessence Publishing Co, Inc; 2010. p. 31–46.
11. Mustarde JC. The correction of prominent ears using simple mattress sutures. Br J Plast Surg 1963;16:170–8.
12. Hollander MHJ, Contini M, Pott JW, et al. Functional outcomes of upper eyelid blepharoplasty: a systematic review. J Plast Reconstruct Aesthet Surg 2019;72:294–309.
13. Hollander MHJ, Schortinghuis J, Vissink A, et al. Aesthetic outcomes of upper eyelid blepharoplasty: a systematic review. Int J Oral Maxillofac Surg 2020;49(6):750–64.
14. Kontoes P. State of the art in blepharoplasty. From surgery to the avoidance of complications. Berlin (Germany): Springer; 2018.
15. Talei B. The modified upper lip lift. Advanced approach with deep-plane release and secure suspension: 823-patient series. Facial Plast Surg Clin North Am 2019;27:385–98.

Moving?

Make sure your subscription moves with you!

To notify us of your new address, find your **Clinics Account Number** (located on your mailing label above your name), and contact customer service at:

Email: journalscustomerservice-usa@elsevier.com

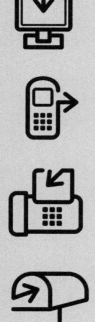

800-654-2452 (subscribers in the U.S. & Canada)
314-447-8871 (subscribers outside of the U.S. & Canada)

Fax number: 314-447-8029

Elsevier Health Sciences Division
Subscription Customer Service
3251 Riverport Lane
Maryland Heights, MO 63043

*To ensure uninterrupted delivery of your subscription, please notify us at least 4 weeks in advance of move.

Printed and bound by CPI Group (UK) Ltd, Croydon, CR0 4YY

08/05/2025

01864724-0018